BS

Charles

thank you

for your

interest

Bill

Charlie

Thank you

for your

Warmt

Bill

Blocked In The USA

The Stem Cell Miracle

The Healing Secret From Medicine's Future That's Saving Lives Today!

By William C. Rader, MD

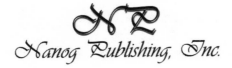

Nanog Publishing, Inc.

Blocked In The USA

Published by

Nanog Publishing, Inc.

3952 Ridgemont drive

Malibu, CA 90265

www.nanogbooks.com

ISBN 978-0-615-32905-5

Dedication

To all the parents who refused to believe the negative prognoses of current medical wisdom and had the courage, hope, and determination to never give up their search to find solutions for their children's illnesses.

Disclaimer

Although I remain unhappy with the possibility of the following declaration resulting in a skepticism regarding the validity of the facts in my book, my lawyers have written the following and insisted that I include the subsequent disclaimer, in order to protect my ability to allow this important medical information to be available to the public. So here it is.

Table of Contents

Introduction 1

It Isn't a Miracle, It Just Looks Like One.............................. 3

Fetal Stem Cell Research in the News.................................... 23

How I Learned About the Stem Cell Miracle.......................... 31

Frequently Asked Questions, Straight Answers 37

Who is Dr. William Rader? 49

My Quest, or Brick Walls and Deaf Ears 65

A Doctor Who Believed 79

Lies, Myths, Misconceptions, and Mice................................. 95

Success Stories: Making the Case for Fetal Stem Cell Therapy 103

In Their Own Words.. 105

Aging and Longevity... 145

AIDS... 157

Alzheimer's Disease.. 167

Autism 175

Bell's Palsy... 197

Brain Damage.. 201

Cancer... 217

Cerebral Palsy... 235

Cirrhosis 261

Coma 265

Cystic Fibrosis.. 269

Down Syndrome.. 273

Eliminate Bone Marrow Donor Registries 277

Epilepsy 279

Heart Disease 297

Infertility 309

Multiple Sclerosis 313

Muscular Dystrophy 323

Parkinson's Disease 331

Sickle-Cell Anemia 345

Stroke 351

My Hope 357

About The Author 361

Introduction

As you read this, the parents of a child suffering from leukemia could be sitting in their doctor's office listening to the devastating news that their child will die in the very near future. The reason? The doctor cannot find a donor match needed to perform a lifesaving bone-marrow transplant.

That child does not have to die.

Right now in my clinic, I have stored in liquid nitrogen the fetal stem cells that could save that child's life—cells with the potential to save the life of virtually every candidate for a bone marrow transplant.

Finding a matching donor is never a problem with fetal stem cells. Because fetal stem cells have no antigenicity, or cellular fingerprint, any fetal stem cell can be transplanted into a patient without harming them or being rejected by their immune system.

Why then must this child die when I have the means to save his life? Why must countless children and adults suffer and die from some of mankind's most devastating diseases when fetal stem cell therapy can improve their condition, prolong life, and in many cases provide a cure?

More than 1,500 of my patients, most of whose cases were considered hopeless, have benefited greatly from fetal stem cell therapy. Yet this treatment is forbidden to patients in the United States.

Why?

Politics, inertia, and ignorance.

Which is to say: the confluence of opposition from drug companies, the United States Food and Drug Administration (FDA), the religious right, and our obstinate medical establishment.

By William C. Rader, MD

Antibiotics changed the paradigm of twentieth-century medicine. Now, in the twenty first century, fetal stem cells can, will, and must become the new revolution in medical care

This book presents case histories and first-person patient accounts of just a few of the cases I have treated with fetal stem cells. I can't possibly discuss here all the disease processes I have treated over the last 15 years. You can find additional information on my web site: www.Medra.com.

This is not just a book about medicine. It is a book about hope.

I write this book primarily for those who have lost hope. For the patient who is told that nothing more can be done. For the parents forced to abandon all hope of recovery for their sick child. I want them to know that fetal stem cell treatment exists. They deserve the right to make choices. Yet current medical dogma forces them to abandon any such hope.

I have been working for years to move the creaky, bogged-down wheels of our inert medical system. Upon reading this book, if you choose to stand with me and help to spread the word, I believe together, we can create an environment where fetal stem cell therapy takes its rightful place in the universally accepted arsenal of weapons used to fight the pain, suffering, and death of millions.

It Isn't a Miracle, It Just Looks Like One

They've been called magic seeds. They have the potential to cure disease, regenerate organs, even prolong life. And they could completely alter the way we practice medicine.

—Fortune magazine [i]

Most probably, your reaction to what you are about to read will be that it is *absolutely impossible* that one treatment modality could produce such incredible positive results for such a wide range of diseases.

If this is your first thought, then consider the following. Pneumonia was a leading cause of death at the beginning of the 20th century. The primary method of treatment was placing a lit candle in a glass on the back of the patient. The resulting survival rate: 2%.

In 1928, Alexander Fleming, a research scientist left his laboratory for a two week vacation, inadvertently leaving behind a culture dish smeared with Staphylococcus bacteria on his laboratory bench, next to an open window. When he returned Fleming discovered mold growing on the dish. The major significance of this discovery was that the mold had destroyed the bacteria in the dish.

The mold was finally recognized for what it was: Penicillin, the most efficacious life-saving drug in the world. Fleming's discovery forever altered the treatment of bacterial infections. Penicillin conquered some of mankind's most ancient scourges, including pneumonia, syphilis, gonorrhea, diphtheria, scarlet fever, gangrene, and meningitis. Many childbirth infections that once killed indiscriminately were suddenly treatable.

Now, imagine a world in which most chronic degenerative diseases can be safely and successfully treated using a new medical procedure that harnesses the intelligence of Creation itself. Imagine a treatment that produces new cells and repairs damaged ones, thereby restoring the human body in accordance with the laws and intents of nature. Imagine a therapy that produces these results:

- An **Alzheimer's** patient is so confused he was unable to find his way home. In a matter of weeks, he reverts to his previous healthy mental state, resuming his activities as dean of a prestigious graduate school and a noted author. His recovery holds fast after five years.
- Potentially provide a **Cure for Leukemia**
- An **AIDS** patient, given only two weeks to live, recovers and returns to a normal life, with no further symptoms of AIDS.
- An **Autistic** child, formerly isolated because of uncontrollable violent behavior, attends a regular school and is better behaved than his "normal" siblings.
- A four year old boy with **Muscular Dystrophy** who has difficulty evening walking easily climbs up 30 stairs the day after his treatment
- Eliminate the need for **Bone Marrow Transplant Registries**.
- A **Diabetic** patient's foot, which had a non healing ulcer, which was resistant to all known medical treatment and therefore would likely be amputated, heals within weeks.

- Reverse the devastating progression of **Myasthenia Gravis**.

- A child with an "untreatable" disease, on life support and declared **Brain Dead** (a complete absence of brain-wave activity) is removed from his life support and eventually returns to a nearly normal life—despite doctors' previous recommendation that the parents "pull the plug."

- A 66-year-old man with alcoholic **Cirrhosis of the Liver** is told that he will die soon unless he receives a liver transplant. Within three months, his liver function is normal, and he is taken off the transplant list.

- An "untreatable" teenager, who was in the "final stages" of **Cystic Fibrosis**, becomes symptom-free and remains so.

- A patient with fatal, untreatable, **Systemic Scleroderma** (a progressive disease that affects the skin and connective tissue) experiences a significant regression of symptoms within three weeks.

- Longevity patients experience strengthening of the **Immune System**, resulting in longer life, marked decrease in the chances of contracting many diseases, including cancer, and significantly increased mental clarity and physical energy.

- A stage 3 (with metastases) **Ovarian Cancer** patient, severely anemic and chronically exhausted, gains the strength to withstand multiple high-dose chemotherapy treatments. Within a month she is highly energetic, has a normal blood count, and has no sign of cancer cells.

- A patient with **Parkinson's Disease** shows marked improvements in gait, voice, balance, shaking, stiffness, and facial features

- A child with **Cerebral Palsy**, who had slurred speech, spasticity, and very limited cognition, achieves significant improvement.

- An **Infertile** woman becomes pregnant after all other efforts available from modern medicine fail.

- A patient's life-threatening chronic **Kidney Failure** is eliminated and remains so after four years.

- After being told she would never walk again, a patient with a **Spinal Cord Injury** regains her ability to walk.

- Symptoms of **Epilepsy** are eliminated in a child who suffered 30 to 40 seizures a day, was taken to several major university neurological centers across the United States, and was treated with 14 various seizure medications—all to no avail.

- A **Brain-Damaged** child, neurologically blind and deaf, is once again able to see and hear.

- A child who suffers constant pain and frequent infections due to **Sickle Cell Anemia** becomes completely symptom-free.

- A **Multiple Sclerosis** patient finds relief not only from her symptoms, but the plaques (scars) in her brain begin to disappear.

- Two and a half years after suffering a **Stroke**, a patient regains normal speech and vision within hours of treatment, and he eventually regains the use of his arms and legs.

- A 14-year-old girl with **Charcot-Tooth Disease** (a progressive and "incurable" nerve and muscle disorder), able to negotiate stairs only by crawling up and sliding down, recovers and can walk and climb normally.

- A child crassly labeled by her doctors as a hopeless **"Vegetable"** becomes interactive with her environment and is clearly seen to experience joy.

- A child with **Down's Syndrome** is transformed into one with a normal physical appearance and higher than average intelligence for his age.

- A 12-year-old child who suffers daily **Migraine Headaches**—with such intense pain and vomiting that he said, "Mommy, I really want to die"—becomes completely pain-free, and the migraines never return.

- A **Cardiac Patient**—who has received all that modern medicine had to offer and still has shortness of breath and sharp chest pain after taking just a few steps—returns to a normal and productive life.

- Eliminate **Genital Herpes** in a patient who had been suffering from painful chronic outbreaks for over 7 years.

- A patient's "untreatable" **Cancer** is eliminated because his body is able to withstand a potently lethal dose of chemotherapy.

The treatment responsible for these apparent "miracles" is Fetal Stem Cell Therapy. All of the cases above are examples from the more than 1,500 patients that I have successfully treated with fetal stem cells.

Does it seem impossible to you that one method of treatment can achieve such dramatic results for such a vast variety of diseases and injuries? If so, please stay with me for at least the next couple of chapters. The science is sound and the results irrefutable. Keep in mind that 150 years ago, established medical science would never have believed that diseases might be caused by creatures too tiny to see.

I am one doctor fighting to be heard above the raised voices of the all-powerful medical establishment, the FDA, and the religious right, who have managed by political action to block even the most basic research into this promising technique.

For the sake of those who suffer, I am desperate to be heard.

I am the only American doctor who has administered fetal stem cell therapy to human patients. The relief experienced by my patients whose conditions were, at one point, declared "hopeless" is the only mandate I need to continue my research until our government comes to its senses.

First, I would like you to consider the science that supports the miracle of fetal stem cells. Then I'll present case histories of individuals with a broad variety of diseases and injuries. My hope is that once you have read their stories, you will ask the same question that is continually on my mind—a question that must be directed to the powerful institutions that control our medical delivery system:

Why is the American medical establishment refusing to objectively evaluate this treatment?

The wheels of American medical research continue to grind ever so slowly. But if you have a loved one suffering from a so-called "incurable" disease, you can't wait years or decades for this therapy to be tested, validated, and approved. The recent change of occupants in the White House provides hope for some progress on fetal stem cell research—something that the Bush administration prevented. Still, under the normal regiment of American medical research and according to conventional medical wisdom, fetal stem cell therapy is still 15 to 20 years from approval. And that doesn't take into account the opposition that emanates not only from some politicians and their fundamentalist constituents, but also from drug companies that stand to lose billions in profits to a more effective non-drug treatment.

And there's one more question you need to ask and perhaps already have: Is Dr. William Rader selling snake oil? Or is he possibly at the beginning of a new pathway in harnessing the healing power of nature?

Before I delve into the science behind fetal stem cell therapy, I'd like to introduce you to someone too young to understand the science, yet far too experienced to doubt it. Her name is Hannah. She is a beautiful, loving child whose inspiring story shows that mankind's healing miracle of stem cells is already upon us—not 20 years away as most "experts" predict.

The Miracle begins…Here's Hannah's story, in her mother's own words:

On May 24, 2003, we welcomed the birth of our third child, Hannah. She was absolutely perfect. She grew and developed normally, even somewhat advanced for her age. She sat up on her own at four months, walked unassisted at 10 months, and was speaking in sentences at 12 months. Hannah was very active and determined to keep up with her two older brothers. She was full of energy, full of life, full of mischief, and full of personality. She began preschool at the age of three, and we watched in amazement as she learned her alphabet, counted to 20, learned to ride a bike, recited her phone number and address, and exuded confidence.

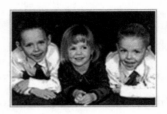

Hannah with her brothers before becoming ill

Then on October 11, 2006, at the age of three and a half years, Hannah's world was suddenly turned upside down. While playing with her grandfather, she tipped over from a sitting position, lost consciousness, and suffered a series of seizures. Grandpa immediately called 911, and she was rushed to the nearby hospital in status epilepticus, a life-threatening condition of repetitive, unexplained seizures preventing the ability to breathe.

She was transported by helicopter to one of the best children's hospitals in our area. Over the next three days in ICU, Hannah underwent a CT scan, which was normal; extensive blood work, which was normal; metabolic testing, which was normal; and an EEG, which was normal. We were sent home with no clear answers as to what had happened to our little girl.

Two days later, the seizures returned and she was transported by ambulance back to the children's hospital and placed on an anticonvulsant called Trileptal. Again she was sent home, but the seizures didn't stop. Within two weeks she was having more than 30 tonic-clonic (or grand mal) seizures per day; atonic drop seizures,

10

causing her without warning to suddenly fall to the ground; more myoclonic seizures than we could count; and repeated episodes of status epilepticus. Her EEG showed global seizure activity, and her frontal lobe was constantly in a seizure state.

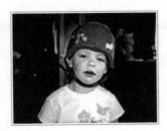

The next three months were a living nightmare for our entire family. Hannah was admitted to the hospital for a total of 41 days in three months with uncontrolled seizure activity. Within three weeks of her first seizure in October, Hannah had lost her ability to speak, to walk, to control her bowels or bladder, and to interact with others. She even lost her ability to recognize Mom and Dad. It was heartbreaking. She would lie in her hospital bed rocking and rolling around on her back, completely nonverbal. She was not engaged in her world.

Neurologists and epileptologists tried in vain to stop her seizures with multiple anticonvulsant medications. We started Hannah on a ketogenic diet, a medically supervised high-fat diet that is sometimes used to treat seizures in children who have medication-resistant severe seizure disorders. While this originally decreased her seizures by about 20 percent, it was not enough to stop them altogether, or to stop the brain damage that was occurring.

In January 2007 she was started on an experimental treatment called intravenous immunoglobulin therapy. Again the initial response seemed promising, but the seizures and resultant brain damage continued.

Eventually we were brought into a small family room at the hospital to discuss Hannah's deteriorating condition. When we entered the room, we were met by two neurologists and a social worker who sat at a table with a box of Kleenex placed in the center. It was clearly evident that the prognosis was very bad.

We were told that Hannah was suffering from idiopathic Lennox-Gastaut Syndrome, a severe and incurable epileptic encephalopathy for which no cause can be identified. My heart sank as her prognosis was described to us. Lennox-Gastaut Syndrome has a 3 to 7 percent mortality rate. It causes severe mental and physical disability. Seventy-eight percent of children with Lennox-Gastaut syndrome will be institutionalized. The associated seizures are intractable to treatment and would continue relentlessly destroying her brain. The prognosis for Hannah was grim. This was a catastrophic pediatric diagnosis.

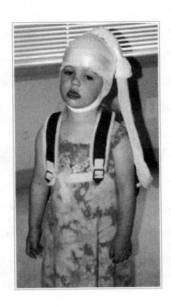

We were completely numb. The facts were in front of us. I asked the doctor if there was any chance that she could recover, or if there was any possibility that the diagnosis was incorrect. The answer was no. Lennox-Gastaut Syndrome is characterized by three distinct features and Hannah had all three. There was no mistake. I cried and hugged the neurology nurse and said, "What do we do now?" Her response will forever be etched in my mind: "Take her home and enjoy her. This is going to get very bad, very quickly."

How could we give up on a child that had so much to offer this world? Was there truly no cause for this disease, or did this simply mean that the cause was yet to be discovered? The answer was clear. If the medical community was certain that there was no known cause for her disease, how then could they be certain that there was no cure? We will never find that which we don't seek.

The goal of Hannah's treatment from the first seizure had been "symptom relief." Seizures themselves are merely the symptom of an underlying problem. If we can't control the symptoms with medication after medication, then the disorder becomes "incurable." We were determined to continue to fight for Hannah's quality of life until no stone was left unturned. Giving up on our child was never an option for us, even when others did.

Endless hours of research through every medical textbook I could access, every medical journal and every internet site I could find, resulted in a connection to an amazing woman named Azita. I learned of Clayton, a young boy who had suffered from Lennox-Gastaut, through a rather obscure magazine article posted on the Internet. Clayton had received fetal stem cell therapy and his seizures had stopped. This was a chance, a stone not yet overturned. I wrote to the newspaper and asked them to forward my information. The magazine agreed, and within a day we received a phone call from Clayton's mom, Azita.

Our sights were set on trying this treatment for Hannah. Of course we were skeptical. It is human nature to question the unknown. I have worked in the health-care field for 18 years, and thus I looked for empirical evidence, clinical reports and the like. There was, however, one distinct problem: There is very little data available on the use of fetal stem cells. The science has been overshadowed by the ethical and religious battle surrounding it.

The next obvious flaw in the traditional system that I had worked within for so long was this: How do you do a double-blind placebo study on a child with Lennox-Gastaut Syndrome? How would you control the variables to make the study meet scientific approval? The answer was

14

clear: Some children would receive a potentially lifesaving treatment, and others, possibly my daughter, would just get normal saline solution. This would be a death sentence for the unfortunate child who received the placebo.

The next question was: How long was the anticipated wait for stem cell therapy clinical trials? I spoke with a cellular biologist and was told that fetal stem cell therapy would likely never be approved in this country, and other forms of stem cell treatments for neurological disorders were most likely 10 to 15 years away. If my daughter was considered mentally retarded within three months of her first seizure, what would be left of her brain in 10 to 15 years, if she was even able to live that long? Children with Lennox-Gastaut don't have the luxury of time. Every day more and more damage is occurring.

The final decision to embark on a journey out of the country was an emotional one, without question. But we promised ourselves and our daughter that we would travel to the ends of the earth and back in an effort to help her.

We did not have the approval of our neurology team. We were told that it couldn't possibly work, that we needed to accept Hannah's diagnosis and prognosis, and that denial was a difficult emotion to overcome.

Our local community rallied around us and raised the funds to send Hannah for her first treatment. When the neurologists learned of the fundraising, they told us, "This money would be far better spent preparing your home and your life for a child with a severe disability." They insisted that there was no scientific evidence to support the claims of Dr. Rader and Medra, Inc.

By William C. Rader, MD

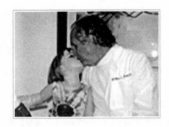

Hannah receiving the Fetal Stem Cells

I asked if they had a great deal of knowledge in regards to his treatment and the answer was this: "No. It can't possibly work; you are wasting your money." What price would be acceptable for my daughter's health and happiness? Hannah was still having multiple daily seizures, at times more than we could count. There was nothing more our doctors could offer. We scheduled her treatment for June 30, 2007.

To our astonishment, 20 minutes after the treatment, Hannah began to roll her head from side to side, and she started to cry. As parents, we learn to recognize the different meanings behind different cries. This one meant that she was scared. She didn't seem to recognize me or my husband. She was pulling away from us and looking around the room as if she was totally lost. I was terrified. My husband took her in his arms and said, "Hannah is okay. You are okay. Daddy and Mommy are here."

She looked at him and said, "Daddy, why did you wake me up?"

We were completely shocked.

My husband and I started to cry, and he asked her, "Where have you been?"

She replied, "I don't know."

Following the treatment, we took her back to our hotel room and waited for the inevitable seizures to strike. No seizures occurred. She had

16

a nap and then independently got out of her bed and started walking toward the bathroom. We scrambled after her, because she was not wearing her helmet and we feared the impending drop seizure. When we asked her where she was going, she looked at us and responded with attitude, "I'm going to the bathroom." Hannah had not had control of her bowels or bladder for over 10 months, and suddenly she was going to the bathroom independently!

After arriving home, Hannah went for 45 days without a seizure. Our doctors were concerned that she was still having regular seizures and that we were just not visualizing them. Hannah was scheduled for a 24-hour EEG in September. The EEG was dramatically improved, and while still irritable, she had no discernible seizure activity in those 24 hours.

We went for a second fetal stem cell treatment in December 2007, and Hannah continued to experience amazing results. She was reassessed by medical professionals and was found to be cognitively age-appropriate, her gross motor skills had improved significantly to only a mild delay, and her speech was accelerated to the 97th percentile.

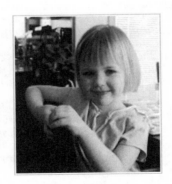

Hannah today

By William C. Rader, MD

Today Hannah suffers from three or four tonic seizures per month during sleep. She no longer has seizures while awake. Hannah is attending a regular public school in kindergarten and is doing very well. She rides a bike, she drives go-carts, she swims, sings, runs, jumps— everything that any five-year-old could and should be doing. Her quality of life has improved 100 percent.

Our daughter is back.

It is totally clear that fetal stem cell therapy changed the course of her disease and gave her back her quality of life and health almost immediately.

Inexplicably, her doctors still do not see stem cell therapy as the cause for her dramatic improvement. However, at least they do admit that they know nothing about it.

The irony of the situation is that we were expected to accept the prognosis for our daughter as described by the neurologists based on their scientific, medically approved testing. EEGs and standardized developmental testing led to the diagnosis. Now she is a normal child again, and the same scientific, medically approved testing that they perform to assess her supports this. The testing procedure did not change. Hannah's condition changed. It is utterly absurd that the same tests that diagnosed her and gave us no hope for recovery are now being dismissed when they show that her condition has dramatically and irrefutably improved.

One day soon, the world will accept what we know to be true. Dr. Rader is a pioneer in the field of stem cell therapy and his work will serve as the basis for stem cell curative medicine in our society. People argue that the clinical evidence is lacking in his research, and that it is providing merely anecdotal evidence. My daughter's EEG is normalizing. This is something that we were told would never occur. We have copies of every EEG report that our daughter has had, and would be happy to share them with anyone who needs clinical proof.

Hannah was assessed by trained medical professionals in the areas of speech, cognitive function, gross motor skills, fine motor skills, and behavior before the first stem cell treatment, between the first and second treatments, and after the second treatment. She has improved to an age-appropriate level in all areas, with the exception of fine motor control. We are confident that with further treatments this too will improve. This is not a mom's interpretation; this is clinical proof that stem cell therapy is effective.

We went to the ends of the earth and back to find something to help our daughter. We found Dr. Rader, and we will be forever grateful for the gift that he has given our family.

Hannah is a normal child, full of life, love and mischief. Our daughter is living her life again.

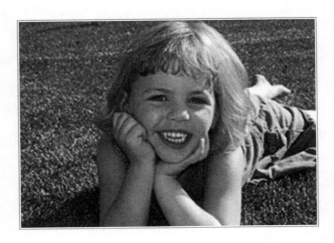

Let me add one more thing to Hannah's mother's profoundly moving account.

The only children in the history of medicine to recover from Lennox-Gastaut syndrome have been my fetal stem cell patients. It has never happened before. And it wouldn't have happened at all under the current system of medical "progress" in the United States.

If you visit my website, Medra.com, you can view the actual video of Hanna's remarkable experience.

As a comparison between what fetal stem cell therapy can accomplish by means of a simple intravenous and subcutaneous administration of fetal cells, as occurred in Hannah's case and what traditional medicine has to offer, I present the following case study of another child with a similar diagnosis. Recently there was a highly publicized "new successful" treatment for a 6 year old little girl who had uncontrollable abnormal seizure activity in one half of her brain. *(Hanna's uncontrollable abnormal seizure activity occurred throughout her entire brain, a much more serious condition).*

The doctors at the University Medical Center told her parents the only way to stop the seizures, which were deteriorating her cognitive function, was through "a radical solution called a hemispherectomy, a daring and complicated over 7 hour surgery in which the neurosurgical team would carefully remove one half of her brain."

She came out of surgery with the left side of her body paralyzed and immediately began intense therapy. Her physical therapy sessions ended three years later.

In a recent interview her parents stated: "We knew that this was our only option to help our daughter, the risk was something that we were willing to deal with because her quality of life was so poor." She was able to return to school, where she is a good student and today she can run and play, although she has a slight limp, wears a brace on her left leg and lost some of her peripheral vision.

(Hanna's complete transformation occurred 20 minutes after receiving the fetal stem cells).

Under current FDA guidelines, scientists would have to first begin studying the effects of fetal stem cell therapy on mice. After perhaps 20 years of animal studies, we might actually be able to commence clinical human trials. Many millions of dollars and much scientific manpower will be wasted on attempting to prove something that has already been proven. Under this regimen, a generation of children, like Hannah, will be deprived of the opportunity to receive this markedly beneficial and sometimes life saving medical treatment.

While the FDA is plausibly the most overcautious and slow-moving medical authority in the world, there is often merit in proceeding cautiously in developing and testing a new drug or therapy. It is important to establish that there are no harmful side effects to new procedures or drugs. However, as explained in the upcoming chapters, it is well established that fetal stem cell therapy has no negative side effects. Nonetheless, the FDA still will not allow us or our loved ones to put our hope in such "unproven" yet promising treatments, even when the certainty of death is staring us in the face.

Innovation and exploration have always been the keys that open the door to new knowledge. In medical research, scientists often get ideas they can't prove, but which are based on previous experience and conscientious research. When the final days, hours, and minutes of human life are ticking away, as was in Hanna's case, isn't it time to take a chance?

The FDA forbids me to give people this treatment.

My own conscience forbids me to withhold it.

If you saw a person drowning, would you throw that person the only life preserver at hand, even if it wasn't a U.S. Coast Guard–approved personal flotation device? Of course you would.

If you believe that we cannot let politics, religious beliefs or bureaucracy deny our God-given right to seek cures for mankind's ailments, then continue reading this book. Consider my work and judge it. Consider the testimonies of parents who never stopped fighting to save their children's lives, even when organized medicine refused further treatment and told them, "Nothing can be done to help your child."

Read the stories, presented here in their own words; of people who were told not only that they or their children had no chance, but that they should not even take a chance on a radical new therapy. These stories are moving and will help you decide for yourself whether or not fetal stem cell therapy can legitimately offer new hope, for the millions who have none.

Fetal Stem Cell Research in the News

Despite all my frustration over my inability to treat patients in the United States, or even see my work examined and evaluated objectively, research on the medical use of stem cells is in fact being conducted.

As I'll soon explain, my first encounter with fetal stem cell therapy took place on a trip to the Ukraine in 1995. A few weeks later, I learned that experiments using fetal stem cells were being conducted by doctors in China as well. I immediately sent an experienced observer to China to bring back all the research data she could find and translate it for me. Sadly, most, if not all, of the individuals involved in stem cell research in the West are unaware of or have ignored previous research conducted in Eastern Europe and China.

News stories reporting research breakthroughs and other major developments in the embryonic and fetal stem cell field are popping up in headlines worldwide. Eye-opening reports about new and exciting studies in the field of stem cell research are emerging just in time to help you judge my work and evaluate the accuracy of what you'll learn from this book about the stem cell "miracle."

Eminent scientists at prestigious universities have validated my work by reporting that they've achieved similar results using fetal and other forms of stem cells in animals that I have with humans. They have proven it in their laboratories, through clinical trials overseen by the National Institutes of Health (NIH). In brief, some of these new reports have revealed:

- **Stem cells can reverse brain defects in mice.** Israeli scientists at the Hebrew University of Jerusalem "have succeeded in reversing brain birth defects in animal models, using embryonic stem cells to replace defective brain cells."[ii]

- **Stem cells could help treat strokes.** A press release from a research sponsor claimed that scientists at the University of Nottingham in the U.K. have replaced stroke-damaged brain tissue in rats. The research tested a process wherein "by inserting tiny scaffolding with stem cells attached, it is possible to fill a hole left by stroke damage with brand new brain tissue within 7 days." A spokesman for the Stroke Association in Britain said of the research findings:

The potential to reverse the disabling effects of stroke seems to have been proved. However the development of stem cell therapy for stroke survivors is still in the early stages and much more research will be needed before it can be tested in humans or used in practice.[iii]

Author's note: We have been successfully treating human stroke patients for over 15 years.

- **Stem cells promote the healing of diabetic ulcers.** A paper was released by a research group at the University of Bristol in the U.K. who "found that fetal stem cells accelerate the closure of ischemic diabetic ulcers, while stem cells from blood of adult donors are ineffective."

The group attributed this finding to the greater ability of fetal stem cells to multiply, to graft onto host tissue, and to repair damaged tissue. According to the release, the researchers reasoned thus:

It is known that wounds heal so well in fetuses that no scar can be visible at birth. It is therefore possible that, when fetal stem cells are transplanted onto diabetic ulcers, they reactivate a fetal program in the recipient to allow those adult ulcers to repair as efficiently as fetal wounds do.[iv]

- **Stem cells may cure some kinds of blindness.** As reported by the Times of India, there's "A ray of hope for the visually impaired! Scientists have made a major scientific breakthrough by developing a stem cell therapy to cure blindness. A team in Britain has developed the treatment which involves replacing a layer of degenerated cells with new ones created from embryonic stem cells to cure age-related muscular degeneration, the most common cause of blindness."[v]

- **NEURAL STEM CELLS GROWN IN THE LAB ARE INFERIOR TO THOSE TAKEN FROM DONATED FETAL TISSUE, UCLA STUDY FINDS:**

Neural stem cells grown from one of the federally approved human embryonic stem cell lines proved to be inferior to neural stem cells derived from fetal tissue.

Researchers from the Institute for Stem Cell Biology and Medicine at UCLA coaxed embryonic cells from the federally approved line, to differentiate into neural stem cells.

A process that might one day be used to grow replacement cells to treat such debilitating diseases as Parkinson's and Alzheimer's.

However, the neural stem cells had an abnormality in a gene called CPT 1A that inhibited expression, a metabolic condition that causes hypoglycemia in humans.

Fan, the senior author said, the study deals with one of the most important aspects in stem cell biology - potential abnormalities in cells derived from human embryonic stem cells.

Stem cells with abnormalities may not effectively treat the diseases they were created to treat, or they may result in secondary problems.

- **Fetal stem cells have a greater potential for fighting cancer than other kinds of stem cells.** Natural killer cells, a component of the immune system, fight viruses and tumors. A University of Minnesota research team, hoping to find a new source of killer cells to boost immunity, hypothesized that natural killer cells derived from fetal stem cells mature much faster than those from umbilical cord tissue; therefore, they would be more effective. Their hypothesis, based upon previous research, was confirmed. According to the head researcher, "We've now proven that these cells are much more potent and effective at killing tumor cells than those coming from other sources like human umbilical cord blood."[vi]

- **Fetal stem cells are more effective than their adult counterparts.** According to research done in Belgium, "Cells derived from…fetal tissues are higher in number, expansion potential and differentiation abilities compared with (stem cells) from adult tissues."[vii]

These recent news stories report astounding scientific results from all over the globe, even though they refer to research still in its infancy. Research in other countries is far more advanced than research here in the United States. According to a recent joint study by Harvard University and the Massachusetts Institute of Technology, Iran is not only involved in embryonic stem cell research; its scientists are actually at the forefront. As reported by the Washington Times:

Controversial in the United States, embryonic stem cell research was embraced in 2002 by Ayatollah Ali Khamenei, Iran's conservative religious leader....(Hassan Ashktorab of the Howard University Cancer Center said), "Policies that may be classified as liberal in the American political system seem to be common sense to Iranian politicians."

Ayatollah Khamenei often cites the Koran's emphasis on preventing human illness and suffering as evidence that stem cell research and Islam are compatible.[viii]

And while the United States may not have approved stem cell therapy, at least one treatment based on stem cells is being tested here. The FDA, apparently sensing which way the wind was blowing, suddenly confirmed—just two days after Barack Obama was sworn in as President—that they've granted approval for a U.S. biotech company to conduct the first human trials using a derivative of embryonic stem cells in hope of reversing spinal cord damage. According to the Associated Press article:

By William C. Rader, MD

A U.S. biotech company says it plans to start this summer the world's first study of a treatment based on human embryonic stem cells—a long-awaited project aimed at spinal cord injury.

The company gained federal permission this week to inject eight to 10 patients with cells derived from embryonic cells...

The patients will be paraplegics, who can use their arms but can't walk. They will receive a single injection within two weeks of their injury.

The study is aimed at testing the safety of the procedure, but doctors will also look for signs of improvement like return of sensation or movement in the legs... (Emphasis added.).[ix]

Omitted from the Associated Press article excerpt above is that the embryos the researchers are using came from the original lines approved by former President Bush. Those embryonic cells were grown with animal products (mouse feeder cells and bovine serum), which necessitates that the patient receive dangerous immunosuppressive drugs to prevent the serious, at times even deadly, graft-versus-host reaction. Further, the embryonic stem cells used were subjected to the addition of chemicals and growth factors to produce oligodendrocytes, a precursor to myelin, which is the insulation of the nerve and the part of the spinal cord that is damaged by the injury. In contrast, I use pristine fetal stem cells, which have nothing added to them. Nor do I give the patient drugs to prevent any type of negative reaction. Pristine fetal stem cells do not cause any such reaction—the body does not recognize them as foreign cells, and therefore the immune system does not attack them. For the same reason, the donor fetal stem cells do not attack the recipient.

Therefore, my patients' immune systems are not weakened by anti-rejection immuno-suppressive drugs, or by any immune reaction to, or from, the fetal stem cells.

My results—96 percent of my 1,500 patients improved, recovering, or healed—speak for themselves. The effect of fetal stem cells is a miracle that awes and humbles me, one that no scientist fully understands. I have spent years studying fetal stem cells and putting them to use in healing human patients. Had I waited for the FDA's approval, I would have achieved little and been responsible for a multitude of people, most of them children, languishing in distress. Many who are alive today would have perished.

President Obama's revised policy signals that the push for eventual victory over the naysayers has finally begun. Capturing the sudden optimism that has gripped researchers worldwide since President Obama lifted the ban on stem cell research, the co-director at the Harvard Stem Cell Institute, David Scadden, made this statement to *Time Magazine*: "It's a wonderful time…. Keep your seat belt on, because this ride is going to be wild."[x]

How I Learned About the Stem Cell Miracle

It ought to be remembered that there is nothing more difficult to take in hand, more perilous to conduct, or more uncertain in its success, than to take the lead in the introduction of a new order of things.

—Machiavelli, The Prince

Given that fetal stem cells are considered taboo in the United States, you might wonder how the enormous potential of fetal stem cell therapy first came to my attention.

It was 1995, and I was in Mexico City. At that point in my career, I had already been the chief psychiatrist for the United States Navy's alcohol program, operated the largest program for bulimia and anorexia in the world, started one of the first HIV/AIDS programs in Latin America, and was conducting clinical research in the prevention of heart disease for a major pharmaceutical company in Mexico City.

At that time, a group of Eastern European doctors had been engaged in research regarding the clinical application of fetal stem cells, and had been trying for over 4 years to get someone in the Western medical community to examine their research... Through a colleague working in Mexico, the doctors heard of this eclectic Dr. Rader and hoped they possibly had found someone who would listen to them.

They were right. I was given a preliminary overview of their work, and the next day I called the two Ukrainian researchers I had been told about. I explained to them that I was fascinated by their research and wanted to meet with them in Kiev. "But with all due respect," I said, "I need to know that you're willing to answer all of my questions, without any reservations." I asked that they also bring a diverse group of the patients in their study for direct and private interviews. Surprisingly, our conversation didn't take very long. Almost immediately, the doctors agreed to my conditions.

Ten days later, I was aboard an Air Ukraine plane. What put me on that plane was the truly astounding notion the Ukrainian doctors had put forward; that fetal stem cells, unlike adult-donor stem cells, have no cellular "fingerprint"—what is called antigenicity. They said that the fetal stem cells neither attack the body's immune system nor are they rejected by it. I thought if this contention turned out to be true, it would count as a major medical discovery.

Here in the United States, leading authorities in the medical community had long suspected that the potential for eradicating innumerable human diseases lay somewhere in the mystery of stem cells. Yet these same experts also believed that the fetal stem cell had antigenicity, and therefore the beneficiary would be subject to a dangerous, sometimes fatal, complication called graft-versus-host disease, in which the donor fetal stem cells attack the recipient.

I had learned something else prior to my departure. These Ukrainian doctors had been able to conduct research that was so controversial in most Western countries because, for better or worse, abortion in Eastern Europe is accepted and common. Therefore, obtaining fetal stem cells was legal.

How I Learned About the Stem Cell Miracle

Although I didn't know it at the time, I was headed on a journey that would put wheels in motion, irrevocably transforming my career and, with any luck, contributing to the future of medicine.

As the airplane approached Eastern Europe, the land of my ancestors, my excitement grew. I like to ask tough questions, but I always keep an open mind, as all doctors should but too often do not. I had asked many questions already on this journey into the unknown and had garnered enough answers to know that meeting these researchers was absolutely crucial. Even before I boarded that plane and left sunny Mexico City, I had a hunch – a powerful one at that. I was tracking a medical miracle, and I felt it was close.

When we landed in Kiev, it was snowing heavily and freezing cold. The doctors picked me up and drove me to their hospital along ice-covered roads packed with tiny old cars, most of them crammed with people. When I commented on that, they joked in English, "You need many people in car to keep warm. Car has no heater." I was thankful that our car did have one.

Within minutes of meeting these doctors, I began peppering them with questions, attempting to get an idea of their experiences with fetal stem cells. The two men gave me startled looks at first, but they came back strong.

"We know your ground rules. We will be telling you everything that you asked for."

We all laughed. And before that 40-minute car ride ended, I began to feel a medical miracle was being born in a most unlikely place.

We arrived at the hospital, and I was surprised to see a building that looked like it had once been in a war zone. We rolled to a stop at a barrier, and a man emerged from a hut to lift it so our car could enter. As we entered the main building, I felt as if I was in a movie set in an earlier era, perhaps World War II. It was dark. The long hallway had only a few bulbs. I soon learned that the electricity often failed completely.

An unusual odor pervaded the building. Everything looked shabby and run-down. I'd never encountered such a hospital. The doctors ushered me into an elevator. It was operated by a woman in a white smock who impatiently gestured for all passengers to board, clanged the doors shut by hand, then turned a brass handle to make the car move. She was clearly in charge of her domain. As we began to ascend, she suddenly barked an order at one of the doctors to move over in order to keep the rickety lift balanced. And he, one of the most important doctors in the hospital, sheepishly shifted his position without complaint.

Moments later the lift stopped, the door opened, and a gurney carrying a corpse was wheeled aboard. No one blinked an eye. This elevator, I later learned, was the only working one in the building, so it served both the living and the dead. And while it's not that unusual to occasionally see a corpse wheeled through the hallways of American hospitals, this poor fellow's bare feet stuck out from under the sheet.

We exited the elevator and passed through another long, dimly lit corridor. I took note of ancient, strange-looking medical equipment. Doctors passing by, like doctors everywhere, had stethoscopes hanging from their necks. Many of the stethoscopes were like the modern devices we see in the Western world, but others looked like antique props from a movie. Finally we passed through double doors into a wing startlingly different from the rest of the hospital. It was modern, clean, and neat. It was as if I had stepped through a time warp, skipping 50 years in a single stride.

You might think I am being unkind in my description of a major Ukrainian hospital in 1995, but that is the reality of medicine in much of the world. For example, according to a U.S. Department of State travelers' bulletin dated October 29, 2008, the American embassy in Kiev "recommends that ill or infirm persons not travel to Ukraine…the level of medical care is not equal to that found in American hospitals." The bulletin warns that, while basic medical supplies are available, "travelers requiring prescription medicine should bring their own. When a patient is hospitalized, the patient, a relative, or acquaintance must supply bandages, medication, and food."

All in all, this seemed an unlikely place in which to discover a modern medical miracle, but good science can flourish anywhere. A big dream, talent, hard work, and luck can take a determined researcher a long way.

My hosts were well prepared. True to their word, they answered every one of my probing questions about their research and methodology backed it all up with medical records and studies that looked valid, and then brought in patients they'd treated. Speaking with these patients through translators was a lengthy process, and some were reluctant to carry on a conversation with a nosy American doctor. But for the most part, things went very well over the next few days.

Astounded by the results I'd seen, I was once again struck by the irony that I was in a nation that could provide only the most primitive medical treatments to their own citizens, yet because of cultural and political idiosyncrasies, these doctors conducted breakthrough research that had the potential to transform the future of medicine.

My mind was still spinning when I boarded the plane to leave Kiev. I am often asked if I learned everything I know about fetal stem cells from them. I always answer: "No, but I wouldn't be where I am today if it weren't for my initial learning experience in Kiev." As a Western doctor, I was hoping to add to their research. By my third trip, I began sharing my own ideas with them, some of which they then integrated into their research program.

As the jet carried me homeward, I knew that I was going to dedicate my life and career entirely to the incredible "miracle" of fetal stem cells.

Frequently Asked Questions, Straight Answers

If you are a candidate for fetal stem cell therapy, or if your child or loved one is, I want you to make your decision based on the best information possible.

Good patients and their advocates are skeptical. They ask questions. They do their best to understand what is happening to their bodies, to understand their disease and why the treatment they are considering might or might not be their best choice.

Here are the major questions that my patients most often ask. The answers deal with the essential political, ethical, and scientific aspects of fetal stem cell therapy.

Why are your clinics overseas?

Because the United States Food and Drug Administration won't let me provide fetal stem cell therapy in America. The FDA requires years of animal studies followed by many more years of double-blind tests on humans before declaring a new therapy or treatment safe and effective. That I have already proven fetal stem cell therapy to be safe and effective makes no difference to the FDA.

The FDA's mandatory studies cost many millions of dollars, take decades to complete, and require giving placebos to patients with debilitating or fatal diseases—people who desperately need this therapy.

Are you the only scientist who believes fetal stem cells can save lives?

By William C. Rader, MD

Absolutely not. There are scientists in other countries who are examining fetal stem cells for possible future clinical use, and also some doctors in the United States have publicly stated that fetal stem cells are the future of medicine.

However, advocating fetal stem cell therapy is difficult in the United States because of all the negative pressure from our deeply entrenched and powerful medical establishment, as well as pharmaceutical companies and religious fundamentalists.

Are your fetal stem cell treatments safe?

There are *no negative side effects* from the fetal stem cells. It bears repeating that, since fetal stem cells have no antigenicity, there is also no risk of graft-versus-host disease.

Also, to ensure the purity and safety of our stem cell material, we test for 14 different criteria, including viral, bacterial, and fungal infections, as well as viability. Moreover, we use PCR DNA testing, which is far more sophisticated and expensive than the screening tests routinely used in the United States for the other stem cell transplants.

As an example, the test routinely used to screen for HIV in the United States is called an Elisa test, or antigen-antibody test. It costs about $30. But the Elisa test can produce false negative readings, showing no evidence of HIV even if the person tested was infected as much as six months to a year earlier. Such false negatives are very rare, but they do happen.

By contrast, our fetal stem cells are checked by what's called a PCR-DNA test, a laboratory process that selects a DNA segment from a mixture of DNA chains, and rapidly replicates it. This creates a large sample of a piece of DNA that is much more suitable for accurate analysis.

Our PCR-DNA test costs $300, not $30. And even if the tissue being tested was infected a week before, our test would register positive for HIV. After the testing in our laboratory is completed, the cells are *double check* then *retested* in Germany, in what is considered to be one of the foremost *✱ 2 lab tests For cell* laboratories in the world.

Why have some medical experts attacked you and questioned your techniques?

Over the last 15 years, I have met with many doctors and scientists, hoping to share my results with the mainstream medical and scientific communities. I was eager to share my research openly, but I was consistently met with indifference and even overt negativity. I'm the only American physician who has treated human patients with fetal stem cells, yet no one wanted to discuss my work. When I tried to approach leading health journalists, they consistently asked me if I had conducted double-blind studies; when I told them I had not, the journalists refused to listen further. I flatly refuse to conduct double-blind studies because they are, to put it bluntly, lotteries. How can we, as modern and civilized doctors, administer fetal stem cells to a child who, for example, is brain-damaged, and give another child suffering from the same condition a placebo of saline solution? One we try to save; the other we allow to continue suffering or to die. How could we so cynically play with human lives? And what better control subject could there be than patients who, in most cases, have tried every available option in mainstream medicine to help them—all to no avail?

By William C. Rader, MD

After years of attempting to share what I had learned, I realized that the entrenched resistance in the worlds of medicine, science, and the media indicated something far more serious than simple apathy or ignorance.

Recent studies show that most Americans favor federal funding for embryonic stem cell research. So why aren't the medical and media elites more eager to inform the public of research conducted in other countries? I do not claim that there is a conscious conspiracy to block stem cell research, but there are several elements within the opposition that, taken together, essentially amount to the same thing. These include the religious right, the fear of losing billions of dollars by pharmaceutical companies, and the political blockage driven by powerful lobbyists for these groups. This is my motive for writing this book. I want to bring this debate directly to you, the public.

David Traver, a stem cell researcher at the University of California, San Diego, and the keynote speaker at an international conference on stem cells, described the present situation well: "Most of what we know about stem cells comes from studying mice, fish and flies."[xi]

We are wasting billions of precious dollars and scientific man-power studying mice in order to prove what has already been proven. Ask yourself this: Instead of conducting endless research trials on mice, why not build on the knowledge gathered in the actual human clinical application of fetal stem cells? Why not jump ahead 20 years right now, using as a basis my clinical experience with more than 1,500 patients?

What about ethical considerations regarding the origin of fetal stem cells?

As a result of original research using a technique that we have perfected (not cloning) in our laboratories, we've been able to successfully multiply fetal stem cells while maintaining their pure, pluripotent state. The results: *one single fetus is able to provide enough stem cell material to treat more than **one million patients***. ✱ 1 Fetus — 1 million patients 1x

One of the main reasons that fetal stem cells are such a controversial issue is that they are derived from aborted human fetuses.

With our newly discovered ability to obtain stem cells for over a million treatments from a single fetus that was destined to become medical waste and instead, we now can relieve the suffering of millions of children and adults. Doesn't that irrefutably change the moral argument?

Instead of fetal stem cells, why not use adult stem cells or stem cells harvested from the umbilical cord?

Adult Stem Cell

Because they are more developed or differentiated, the other forms of stem cells do not have nearly the potent healing power of fetal stem cells.

Since fetal stem cell research has been essentially banned in the United States, scientists have settled for conducting research on other types of stem cells, such as: allogenic (adult donor), autologous (from patients themselves) and stem cells taken from sources as diverse as fat, placenta, the foreskin of a newborn's penis, the umbilical cord, hair follicles, amniotic fluid, the nasal membrane, breast milk, skin and menstrual discharge.

Fat
placenta
foreskin
umb. c
hair f
Amnio
Nasal
mens
breast
skin milk

Furthermore, an extremely important and significant difference between fetal stem cells and all other stem cells is that pristine neuronal stem cells can be isolated from the brain tissue of the fetus. There is no other source of pure, pristine neuronal (nerve) stem cells. Some researchers working with mice are still trying to create a form of a neuronal stem cell by adding substances such as neuronal growth factor to undifferentiated embryonic stem cells. The result: a very limited number of attenuated neuronal stem cells, which lack the purity and efficacy of fetal neuronal stem cells.

Fetal stem cells are "pluripotent free agents." That means they are the only cells (besides the limited number of eggs within a fertile woman's ovary) that contain the entire "database" of the human body.

They have the capacity to become any of the body's 220 cell types. In simple terms, what you need is what you get.

Also, other kinds of stem cells have antigenicity, a "cellular fingerprint" that can cause the dangerous, sometimes lethal rejection phenomenon of graft-versus-host disease. When adult donor (allogenic) stem cells, or stem cells derived from umbilical cords, are used, they can require immunosuppressive drugs to prevent rejection. And because these drugs suppress the immune system, they leave the patient highly vulnerable to serious infections and diseases. Fetal stem cells are not antigenic—that is, they do not contain a cellular fingerprint—so the patient's immune system does not recognize and attack them as foreign invaders, nor do the fetal cells attack or harm the recipient. Consequently, contrary to generally accepted medical opinion, nothing is required to prevent rejection—such as an immunosuppressive drug, steroid, or antihistamine.

Here is another reason fetal stem cells are superior to other forms of stem cells: these older cells lose the length of their telomeres and produce less and less telomerase, an enzyme that creates the telomere. A telomere is like a protective arm at the end of a chromosome that protects cells from injury. As we age, telomeres become shorter and shorter, leaving us more vulnerable to aging and disease. The telomeres of fetal stem cells, in contrast, are at full strength.

Imagine a knight whose lance is worn down a bit in every battle. As time goes by, it becomes harder for him to defend himself and easier for his enemies to penetrate his defenses and knock him off his horse.

It's not that adult and umbilical cord stem cells, for example, cannot achieve positive results. But those results pale in comparison to what fetal stem cells can accomplish.

I have treated patients who had received adult or umbilical cord stem cells with minimal to no effect. After administering the fetal stem cells, these patients' conditions consistently improved.

How do the neuronal fetal stem cells actually work to bring about healing?

Once neuronal fetal stem cells are administered to a patient subcutaneously (under the skin), the cells migrate via the lymphatic system, cross the fat-soluble blood-brain barrier, and then enter the central nervous system—the brain and spinal cord. These neuronal fetal stem cells then find the damaged areas and carry out their reparative functions.

43

By William C. Rader, MD

What is the role of the Hematopoietic (blood forming) fetal stem cell?

Hematopoietic fetal stem cells are programmed to protect the fetus as it develops into a complete human being. Their function, besides having the ability of becoming any of the 220 cell types of the body, is to [create organ systems,] as well as [repair damaged cells and tissues.] They have the innate ability to navigate directly to the problem area and then rejuvenate or repair the pathology. So when they are transferred intravenously, or into the bloodstream of a patient, they function the same way—as if that patient were a very large fetus that needed there care and protection.

As I explained earlier, the fetal stem cells contain full length telomeres, which provide the recipient the greatest protection. As you get older, your immune system naturally weakens. When the fetal stem cells are administered, they [improve the immune function] in patients by at least 10 times, greatly reducing the chances of getting the flu, or even cancer. That doesn't mean the person will never get sick, of course, but the odds are greatly reduced. Look at it this way: what percentage of 8 year olds have cancer compared to 60 year olds? The difference being the relative strength of their immune systems.

Wouldn't it be wonderful to get a brand-spanking-new immune system as you reach middle age, one that is even stronger than an 8 year old's immune system?

Once administered, fetal stem cells multiply rapidly at a controlled rate and continue to bolster your health for a lifetime. And while they generate this brand new, very strong immune system, they also support the activity of your native immune system. Fetal stem cells

44

not only replace and rebuild damaged tissue; they also release trophic (growth) substances called *cytokines* that stimulate dormant cells and speed up the repair of cells, tissues, and organs.

What do I mean by "dormant cells"? When a part of the body is damaged, some tissues that appear to be destroyed may actually just be merely dormant. These tissues can potentially be restored to normal function. Unfortunately, no current laboratory test that can determine if such tissues have been destroyed or are merely dormant, awaiting a "miracle" to revive them.

Waking up these dormant tissues and cells is a very important role of the *cytokines* in fetal stem cell therapy. Their effect can be immediate, restoring measurable function even within one hour of administration.

You have read the story of Hannah, who experienced incredible improvement a mere 20 minutes after she was treated. That is not an isolated phenomenon.

A further dramatic example of the immediate effect of the *cytokines* occurred in two cardiac patients we treated using a recent method I developed. They had suffered severe heart failure and could take only a few steps before suffering shortness of breath and sharp chest pain. They had sought out all available help for their condition, but modern and alternative medicines failed to provide them any relief.

We performed a benign procedure no more invasive than a routine angiogram, injecting fetal stem cells directly into certain areas of their hearts. Within **30 minutes of the treatment, their heart function increased by an average of 60 percent, as measured by ejection fraction studies (a measure of cardiac output). Both patients went**

back to living basically normal lives and have maintained these improvements up to this writing, two and one half years later.

This data is backed up with the case studies and computer readouts.

The paragraph above is in bold type so that you can find it easily and, if you choose, show it to your own physician or cardiologist.

Chances are he'll tell you it is completely impossible.

Here's another example of the immediacy of the cytokine effect: A brain-damaged four year old boy, unable to stand on his own, was brought to my clinic by his parents after they had tried many therapies without success.

As you may know, it's a commonly accepted medical "fact" that that there is no known treatment that can significantly and permanently reverse severe brain damage.

Forty five minutes after he received the fetal stem cells, his mother was holding him sitting on the floor, when he suddenly stood up, walked out of his mother's arms, and began to walk around the room. Even when he almost tripped, he quickly regained his balance. Every person in the room began to applaud, with tears in our eyes. And that little boy began to laugh and clap his hands right along with us. That is a moment I will never forget.

Another example of the cytokine effect involved a high-ranking police officer who came to me two years after a debilitating stroke left him weak and barely able to move his left arm and leg. His speech was slurred and his vision was significantly impaired. He was a tough cop, determined to do anything he could to regain his strength and the use of his limbs.

As he was receiving the fetal stem cells, his speech and vision began to normalize. He actually became upset, thinking we'd given him the wrong cells because his greatest hope was to regain function in his arm and leg. I explained to him that that would happen in time as well.

A few months later, the officer indeed regained the use of both limbs. Eventually, his condition returned to almost normal, and he went back to work as a full-time police executive, even occasionally leaving his desk to work in the field.

The immediate improvement in this patient's speech and vision is a perfect example of how swiftly and efficiently fetal stem cell cytokines can arouse dormant areas of the brain.

As a reminder, these remarkable results were achieved two years after the officer's stroke. Imagine what might have happened if he had been treated with the fetal stem cells immediately!

Who is Dr. William Rader?

When I wrote the original draft of this book, I kept any personal information about myself at a bare minimum because I was concerned it might distract from what was truly important: the significance of fetal stem cells as a major new medical breakthrough.

Subsequently, I was convinced by friends—several of whom are successful authors and publishers—and also, most importantly, by my wife Debra, that you, the reader, should clearly understand how I evolved into becoming the singular advocate for the clinical use of fetal stem cells.

Therefore, I will attempt to explain how "Little Billy Rader" became Dr. Rader. In actuality, there was always Dr. Rader in "Little Billy Rader" and today there is definitely "Little Billy Rader" in Dr. Rader.

The answer to what put me on the path to becoming Dr. Rader, I believe, lies in my childhood. Even as a child, I marched to a drummer no one else seemed to hear.

I grew up in Brooklyn, New York. I was a skinny little Jewish boy in a neighborhood where just about everybody else was Jewish.

I was an unusual kid. I had my own unique perspective and used my individual judgment to make decisions. It wasn't that I was trying to be different; I just had a way of doing things and arriving at solutions by methods that even I can't explain cogently.

My older brother, a good kid but mischievous, was always getting into typical kid trouble. I never did. I was quiet, never overtly drawing attention to myself. I guess I was a strange kid, but I just never saw the point of doing things that I absolutely knew, in advance, were going to get me in trouble. It's not that I was a goody-two-shoe. I just didn't care about proving myself to anyone, especially by being macho or "raising hell."

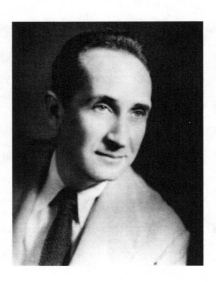

My father was a respected businessman, loved by just about everyone he ever came into contact with. He owned the Rader Drug Company, a financially successful wholesale drug business, which he had always hoped I'd eventually take over.

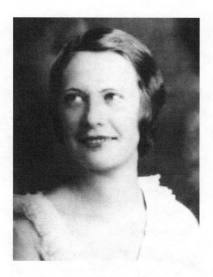

And my mother? My mother loved me unreservedly. She was as beautiful as a movie star, and her soul was even more beautiful. She lived in very good physical and mental health to the age of 99 because she received the fetal stem cells. I believe she would have lived even longer had her doctor not made a tragic clinical error.

My impulse to help others was always there inside me, even as a child.

By William C. Rader, MD

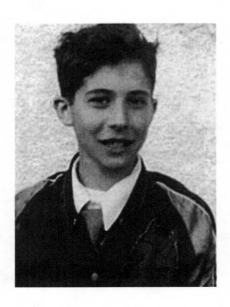

When I was eleven years old, I came home from the movies one day, eating my favorite deli treat: a big, juicy kosher pickle from a barrel, what we called in those days a "nickel pickle." Suddenly I saw a commotion out in front of a neighbor's house. A car was stopped at a strange angle in the street, and a police car was parked behind it. I went over to see what was going on. There were two big Irish cops dealing with an automobile accident, asking people what they'd seen. I was just a kid, so nobody paid any attention to me when I started walking around, checking everything out. I was always walking right into the middle of things. I once walked between two grown men who were about to come to blows. I yelled, "Stop this now!" It broke the tension between them, and they both laughed at the crazy kid. It's not that I'm particularly brave. My curiosity simply overwhelms fear or any other emotions I might have at the time.

Anyway, a crowd gathered on the sidewalk near this accident, and everyone was arguing and making a lot of noise. Some of them kept pointing toward a neighbor's house. So I walked over and went into the neighbor's house. In the front of the house was a sunroom where a woman was lying on a couch, whimpering. She was all alone and obviously very pregnant. I walked over to her and asked her what was going on. She explained, "I was coming down the street, a car crossed in front of me, so I hit the brakes and my stomach hit the steering wheel, and then the police came, and …Oh, God, I hope my baby is okay."

I just looked at her very calmly, and said, "Ma'am, my brother is going to go to medical school. Please be very quiet for a minute, and let me check you out." That was not a lie, by the way. It probably sounded to her like my brother was already in training to be a doctor. He was in high school at the time, but he was definitely headed on to medical school (he is a doctor today).   I kept shushing the woman as she tried to speak, calmed her a bit, then put my ear to her belly and listened very intently. After a long moment, I looked at her and nodded. "Everything is okay," I told her. "Everything is going to be fine."

I may have instinctively believed that this woman and her baby were in no danger, but of course it was essential for her to be evaluated by her doctor. Well, she calmed down. She was fine for a few moments. Then, all of a sudden, she started whimpering again, but this time louder.

I asked her, "What is it? What's the matter now?"

I'll never forget the look on her face when she said, "My husband is going to kill me."

"What are you talking about?"

She grew nearly hysterical, explaining that her husband had told her he didn't want her driving the car while she was pregnant. "When he finds out that I was driving and got into an accident, he'll beat me up."

She looked very frightened and covered her face as if already ducking her husband's blows.

I told her she had to remain calm for the baby's sake. Then I said, "Don't worry about your husband. I'll handle it."

So I went over to one of the officers and kept tugging at his sleeve until he paid attention.

"Kid, we're busy here…beat it," he told me. But even as a youngster, I was pretty hard to ignore. I told the cop and his partner, "This is a pregnant lady and she needs to be calm, but she's really scared that her husband is going to beat her up. She could lose her baby if you don't help."

After talking to the two cops, it turned out there had been no harm done in the accident, and the woman was free to go.

I told them, "Okay, this is what I think you should do." I pointed at the first officer and said, "You drive her in her car and stop about a block from her house." I pointed at the other officer and said, "You follow them in your police car. Let her drive the last block to her house. That way, her husband won't know anything about the accident. You got it?"

Believe it or not, both of those big Irish cops nodded like it was a fine idea. They were listening to me like I was a grownup. I went back to the woman and told her what was going to happen. She was relieved, calmed down, and then thanked me.

Then in a very clear and firm voice I told her, "You and your baby are fine, but you must do what I am about to tell you. I have done all this for you. Now you have to do something for me. As soon as you get home, call your doctor. Tell him what happened. And then I want you to see him today." And then in an even louder and more forceful voice I said; "Will you promise me?"

She promised

"For sure, you will see him today?"

She nodded in agreement.

I walked her to her car and helped her in the passenger side. I then went over to the other side of her car to the officer who would be driving. I started going over the plan, reminding him of the details – acting like he was the 11-year-old, not me.

Our role reversal was strange for a number of reasons, including the fact that even though he was sitting, I had to stand on my toes to keep my head even with his. All three of them waved goodbye to me then took off.

When I got home, I told my mother what had happened. And even though my fabulous mom adored me, she was concerned about what I had done, acting like an expert and all. I suppose what I did was a pretty outrageous assumption of authority for a kid. When my father came home and my mother told him the story, he listened carefully and finally said, "You did good son. I'm very proud of you." Eventually my mother also agreed that, although it was unusual behavior for an eleven year old, I had done the right thing.

As a child, others tended to treat me like I was a "little genius", or just an "arrogant asshole." Most commonly it was the latter.

When I was in my teens, I sat down with my parents and told them: "I'm thinking of becoming a doctor." They didn't overtly object but reminded me that our family's very successful business would someday be mine. My father also rightly pointed out the practicality that just because you want to be a doctor doesn't necessarily mean you can become one. The rigors of getting the proper grades, as well as the extreme competition for becoming accepted to medical school required serious consideration. After careful thought, I decided I would give being in the family business a try. So in college, I earned my degree in business administration. After graduation I started working at the Rader Drug Company, but it totally bored me. It held no challenge. I began to languish mentally.

Then one day I realized I made a mistake and had no choice but to pursue my dream of becoming a doctor.

Two weeks after that epiphany, I decided to test out the possibility of becoming a doctor. Because I was a resident of New York, I flew to the State University of New York at Buffalo Medical School and went to the office of the dean of admissions. I explained to his secretary that although I did not have an appointment, I was hoping to have a few minutes of his time.

He agreed to see me, and we spent the next hour discussing what I would have to complete, academically, with top grades, in undergraduate courses before I could even submit my application. As I had no pre-med courses in my previous college education, he said it would require two years to complete. I asked if I could accelerate the process by taking all of the requirements in a school year and a summer. Since I would have to take 101 (first year courses) and 102 (second year courses) at the same time, he informed me that he would not give me any latitude in my grades.

When I left his office, I told him if he allowed me to be a medical student, he would one day be proud of his decision. I said that believing that I would be a caring and dedicated doctor, one he would be proud of. I had no idea I would become a "known" doctor.

Subsequently, I left the Rader Drug Company, with my parents' support, and moved to Buffalo to start undergraduate school in time for the very next semester.

My abilities as a student were less important than my determination to be a doctor. There were over 300 other pre-med undergraduate students, most of who were away from home for the first time and were more interested in partying than studying. Since we were graded on a curve, there were only three others I had to worry about. They had little plastic holders in their shirt pockets filled with multiple pens and pencils and slide rulers attached to their belts at all times. (It was the early sixties and there were no PC's at that time).

One year and one summer later, I was admitted to medical school. Receiving that letter was one of the most exciting and significant moments of my life.

Now to my experience in medical school. Instead of "keeping my head down" and keeping quiet like the other students, I was always poking it up and questioning things. I remember one incident that didn't make me very popular.

I was attending a lecture in neurology in one of those old style class-rooms that you see in the movies, with ascending levels of seating that look down on the stage where the professor lectures.

That day, they'd wheeled in a patient who was in really bad shape; twisted, bent over, drooling. The head of the department of neurology was in charge of the lecture. Without even introducing himself to the patient, he started poking this poor man with pins, vibrating tuning forks, and a rubber hammer. At the same time he was lecturing to us about how impulses transmitted from the brain can reach places where certain fibers cross, and knowing all the different places where they cross is how you can eventually locate the lesion, and...blah, blah, blah.

So the professor's playing "Where's The Lesion?" and I'm not very interested because I was anxiously waiting to find out how we can help him. The other medical students were very excited. Shouting out: "Oh, yeah, because it's here . . . so it's crossed there, so the lesion is probably either there....or below when the nerve fibers crossed back again."

And here's an important point: even though the patient was twisted and bent because of errant brain activity, mentally he was able to comprehend everything that was happening to him, like, being poked and prodded with implements by a pompous professor before a gawking crowd of students. Well, eventually they pinpointed the lesion's location. Now I thought, finally we were going to discuss his treatment.

It was at this point the Professor waved at his assistant to wheel the poor fellow away. The professor called out, "Next patient!"

I jumped out of my seat and shouted, "But what can you do for him?" The other students started groaning: "Oh, there goes the pain-in-the-ass Rader again!"

So what did the professor say – right in front of this tortured man? "Rader, there is nothing that can be done." His cold response crazed me. I shouted back: "Then why did we put him thru this painful and emotionally humiliating experience? Why not try just holding him in your arms and explain to him about how new medical interventions in the future might possibly help him? Try to understand what he must be going through. Because he's hearing me right now — and he's hearing you right now!"

Oh, that encounter got me in big trouble. But I didn't care. To me, it was a simple question: What is the function of a neurologist? What do they do, in terms of helping patients? Neurologists can spend a great deal of time and money just on diagnosing. And then in many cases they end up informing the patient that nothing can be done for them. Obviously many times, they can help patients with medications, but all too often these drugs also can have serious side effects. I'm not suggesting by any means that most patients can be cured – but every patient can be helped and comforted, even by a simple, kind remark that shows they're still respected as a human being, not some defective creature.

I remember touring a mental institution during college, back in the days when they didn't have drugs like phenothiazines, or similar major tranquilizers. There were truly frightening mental wards where people were crawling around on the floor or ran around banging into walls, with feces literally dripping from their diapers.

As our group walked into one of these wards that day, a blind adolescent suddenly scurried toward us on his hands and knees, drooling and grunting. The stench from his diaper was shocking, and everyone gasped and backed up as he approached. But I just stood there. He found me and then actually crawled up on me. So I held him. I said comforting words to him and then I kissed him. So why did he choose me, rather than another in the group? Since he was blind I don't believe it was because I was the closest to him.

I could be wrong, but I would like to think he sensed my empathy. And even though I wasn't yet a doctor, and couldn't treat him medically, I feel I gave him a moment of comfort.

As I am writing this, I'm concerned that it sounds like it's all about me, the superhero, and how wonderful and empathetic I am, instead of my agenda to convey an example of how anyone can give comfort to someone who is mentally or physically "different", creating even a slight positive change in their life, instead of just turning away.

The initial connection you make with a patient can be the beginning of healing. Studies indicate that showing a patient you're truly concerned and committed to them can actually improve their ultimate outcome.

As I alluded to at the beginning of this chapter, the "Little Billy Rader" who helped the pregnant woman, is fundamentally the same as Dr. Rader. The main difference is simply their age.

As a source of income during my internship and residency, in the evenings and on weekends when I wasn't on duty at the hospital I ran the emergency room for the Pasadena California Police Department and rode their ambulance.

One night, the police department called me out to an extremely dangerous street situation. A psychotic man had locked himself inside his car with his small child and wife. The man had his son in his arms, gripping him so tightly that the child was beginning to turn blue.

The car was surrounded by squad cars and an army of cops. The officer in charge told me they knew the man to be dangerous because when they'd encountered him on a previous occasion, he'd gone absolutely berserk and took down five cops — even though they were trying to control him with their nightsticks.

He said that they had tried everything to get him to release his child or even to just lessen his grip on the boy, but the closer they would get to his car to attempt to talk to him, the tighter his grip would become.

It looked to the officer like the child was struggling to breath and could even possibly die because his father was squeezing him so tightly. At this point, fearful for the child's life, the officer told me as a last option that they were now seriously considering shooting him.

I told the head officer: "The man is psychotic; therefore that makes this a medical emergency. I am the doctor. So I'm in charge — not you. Take your policemen out of sight right now. Go around the corner so that he can't see you, and I'll deal with him." He seemed almost relived to relinquish responsibility for the situation and ordered his men to withdraw, but of course they were observing covertly.

I felt the reason he was holding his child so intently was to protect him from the police, who he feared because of the major altercation he had with them in the past.

I walked back to the car and knocked on the window and said, "Hi, I'm Dr. Rader. Do you know who I am? Do I look familiar to you?" (At that time, I was a known medical expert on television).

I don't know if he actually recognized me, but with this new energy of calm and friendliness rather than fear and aggression, he started to calm down and eased his grip on his son. I engaged him in conversation, attempting to keep his attention and gain his trust. After awhile I told him it was difficult to hear him and could he please roll down the window. He finally agreed and opened the window. I leaned in the open window and said: "That is the cutest little boy. Is he your son"? He nodded his head. I looked over at the mother who was still crying and gave her a stern look and told her to be quiet. At that moment, I quickly reached through the window, opened the door and slid in right next to him.

I looked directly at him and asked if I could hold his boy, "I'd love to hold your son." He actually loosened his grip even more as I kept talking to him, while at all times looking him directly in the eye. Finally he allowed me to hold his child. I continued to ask him questions as I handed the boy over to his mother.

Eventually, he became even more relaxed and began answering my questions. I found out what had happened – he'd been on medication, but had stopped taking it, and as I had thought, being unable to think clearly, he found himself surrounded by the police and became terrified for himself and his family.

I told him: "Being off the medication has made you very fearful and paranoid. You know, you're in control and do not act crazy when you are on medication. But now because of your behavior, the cops are crazed. They may shoot you, because they're afraid of you – remember what happened last time you confronted them? I know you would never hurt your son, but they are afraid that it could happen. It's lucky they didn't shoot you before I arrived."

This was a big, scary looking guy, and I was sitting just an arm's -length away from him. But I seem to do very well with "crazy" people. They appear to sense that the "Little Billy Rader part of me isn't afraid of them and that Dr. Rader isn't going to hurt them.

So I looked him directly in the eye and said: "Look, here's the deal. Right now as I said, the police are fearful and crazed. Now this may sound strange to you, but I'm going to walk away for a minute, I'm going to get some handcuffs…and handcuff you. Because if I don't take you out of this car in handcuffs, they'll be thinking you might hurt me, or whatever — and they may shoot you. So will you do this for me?"

He nodded his head in agreement. I turned to the mother and told her to sit there quietly with her child and that I would be right back.

I got out of the car and looked back at him. He was sitting calmly. I walked around the corner where the police were, got a pair of handcuffs from the officer, asked him for the keys, and then reminded him to keep his men out of sight.

When I got back to the car, I sat beside him again and told him I was sorry I had to handcuff him but it was the safest thing to do for all of us, including his son. He understood and allowed me to handcuff him.

When we got out of the car, there wasn't a cop in sight. We walked over to the ambulance. I put him inside, removed his handcuffs and off we went to the hospital. Once there, I gave him an injection of a major tranquilizer, and he was released a few hours later.

While we were in the hospital, he committed to me that he would keep taking his medication without fail. I do not know for sure if he kept his word, but I do know that over the next 3 years I worked at the Pasadena Emergency Center, the police kept track of him and there was never another incident.

This behavior on my part is seen by most everyone as me being stupid, acting very dangerously, crazy…or all three.

I would imagine you agree with them. But I believe an edge is a ledge for me. What I mean by that is: because of my apparent insight into and understanding of people and their behavior, I seem to be able to correctly evaluate situations quickly and then act accordingly. What is standing on a tiny dangerous edge for others is, for me, standing on a safe wide ledge. Right or wrong, I believe I connect especially well with those who are frightened or even psychotic.

When I was a psychiatric resident, besides working for the Pasadena Police Department, I was administratively in charge of the largest psychiatric hospital in Southern California in the evenings and weekends. One of my responsibilities was; if one of the psychiatric resident employees failed to show up, I would have to assume his duties.

In the middle of one particular night, when I was on replacement duty, I was sleeping in the psychiatric hospital's doctor's quarters when I was suddenly awoken by someone standing over me. After seeing who it was, I remember feeling relieved that it was just a schizophrenic patient rather than some neurotic intruder.

With all the above verbiage, I'll bet you still think I'm going to get myself in "deep trouble" someday. Perhaps you're right.

My Quest, or Brick Walls and Deaf Ears

All they could see are the problems and the fears, but none of the potential. They are committed to the fact that this is the way it is, and that is all you can expect. If you have a vested interest in the ongoing game, you are frightened by anything that might change it.

—Dr. Richard Alpert (Baba Ram Dass)

If you have not heard of my work until now, it isn't because I've tried to keep it a secret.

Over the years, I have tried very hard to make my research public and to find ways to treat patients in this country. Time and time again, I have wound up talking to a brick wall.

Under our nation's current medical system, scientists and researchers who rock the boat by trying to promote radical research, unconventional therapies, or by challenging the system's economic structure do not fare well. They find themselves cut off from traditional sources of funding, fired from their positions at scientific institutions and research centers, and facing sanctions from peers and scientific organizations.

This, in fact, is a very old story.

Four hundred years ago, Galileo, the father of modern science, argued that the earth was not the center of the universe, but rotated around the sun. Forced to defend himself before the Roman Inquisition against capital charges of heresy and under threat of torture, Galileo recanted his theory, publicly stating that the Earth remained stationary at the center of the heavens. According to legend, he then muttered, "And yet it moves." He spent the rest of his life under house arrest, and his book on heliocentrism was banned.

By playing it safe, scientists and researchers help to maintain the medical status quo while suppressing bold, innovative research that could yield new treatment for millions. Why? One reason is that the huge companies that market pharmaceuticals and other medical therapies and supplies are happy to fund research that yields profits to them; these companies are not so pleased about research that could render great numbers of profitable drugs outdated. And of course, researchers engaged in long-term, well-funded projects are reluctant to support discoveries that would render their studies obsolete before they are completed.

Sadly, even scientists working in embryonic stem cell research are guilty of the play-it-safe-and-slow approach. They conduct research on mice. According to their own published timetable, human use is most likely 20 years away. And even though they know what my colleagues and I have accomplished, many perpetrate a bold-faced lie when they publicly state that the fetal stem cells we are using have antigenicity and therefore are not only potentially harmful, but could even be life-threatening.

I have 1,500 patients who prove otherwise—patients who were given no medication to protect them from antigenicity and yet experienced no negative reaction.

My Quest, or Brick Walls and Deaf Ears

I would like to share with you some of my experiences in trying to bring fetal stem cell therapy to the United States.

As a prime example of the entrenched, stubborn, vocal resistance to fetal stem cells on the part of doctors and researchers, I give you Dr. Evan Snyder. Dr. Snyder is Program Director for Stem Cells and Regenerative Medicine at the Burnham Institute for Medical Research in La Jolla, California. He is also an Independent Ethics Advisor to Stem Cell Authority Ltd., a company publicly traded on NASDAQ in the business of collecting and preserving umbilical cord stem cells. Although Dr. Snyder's research is restricted only to mice, he is considered one of our nation's leading stem cell researchers.

Dr. Snyder is well aware, in great detail, of every aspect of my work—how we isolate, prepare, test, and retest our fetal stem cell material, how we administer it, and my successful results.

I have had several conversations with Dr. Snyder over the last few years, as have some of my patients. Both the patients and I provided him detailed information about my program and openly answered all his questions. Yet after having received all this information, Dr. Snyder has publicly stated: "I am skeptical of anyone who goes straight to patient's off-shore and does not publish animal data first and then go through rigorous screening in this country to conduct a proper clinical trial. I regard them as intellectually weak and reckless at best, and cowards and exploiters at worst. Until they are published in a peer-reviewed mainstream journal, they do not exist."[xii] Dr. Snyder has even said, "What Doctor Rader is doing is horrific. He is a used car salesman selling snake oil."

Why would Dr. Snyder say these things? Look at it this way: What would happen to Dr. Snyder and other outspoken leading mice researchers if my clinical experience became widely known? Who would be interested in what happened to a mouse once they had examined my results with over 1,500 human patients? What would happen to these researchers' positions, research facilities, and millions of dollars in grants? I cannot see into Dr. Snyder's heart, but I can think of no other motive for these detrimental statements.

Here is another example of the resistance I have faced. I met with one of the top science writers in the United States, hoping to interest him in my work. The meeting was arranged by his boss, a social acquaintance of mine and the editor of a highly respected newspaper. I went into the interview, feeling very positive. I had just concluded an all-out effort to share my fetal stem cell research with American medical experts, and it hadn't gone well. But my optimism rested on the expectation that this highly regarded science writer was a tough, objective journalist who cared only about digging for the truth, unlike my overcautious medical colleagues.

I was excited to explain the research path I had taken after discovering the medical advances made in the Ukraine. I told him how I had established a hospital and clinics abroad, helped pioneer new medical techniques, and achieved positive results with fetal stem cell treatments on, at that time, more than 1,000 patients—many deemed hopeless or terminally ill.

The journalist immediately responded that he was not interested in testimonials. These were all anecdotal case histories, he said. My patients were just saying that they'd been helped and even cured. Why had I never performed double blind studies on my patients according to the established scientific method, or published my work in peer reviewed medical journals?

I told him that I knew from multiple case histories that my treatment method could save a child's life. A child who was deemed to be "untreatable" and I had no intention of killing a child just to satisfy someone's intellectual curiosity. What if it was his child who received the placebo? How would he then feel about the so-called scientific method?

He began to aggressively attack my position, and I realized I was possibly creating an enemy, but I persisted. I asked as a prominent scientific journalist, did he not have the responsibility to check out my exposition and establish whether I was telling the truth?

I argued: "If what I'm saying is true, you could help save countless lives. And if it's not, you could write a story exposing me as a crook and charlatan. Here's my proposition: I'll allow you to choose any patients I've treated, and I'll bear all expenses to bring them here to you. You can question them thoroughly, with no interference from me, because I won't even be there." The reporter flatly refused. He repeated that he wasn't interested in testimonials and then ended the meeting.

It is astounding to me that people such as this journalist can't see that research carried out by "unconventional" means can, at times, also have significant merit. I offered him every chance to expose me as a fraud. If I were scamming hundreds of desperate people, charging them thousands of dollars to leave the United States for bogus treatments, wouldn't that make a compelling story?

Ironically, my adult patients and the parents of the severely ill children do exactly what I was asking the journalist to do: They examine all the facts objectively and in detail. It isn't unusual for me to have multiple conversations over several months with the parents of a sick child, and to field many sophisticated questions from them, before a final decision is made. They are acting with appropriate due diligence and exercising healthy skepticism.

You would think researchers would beat a path to my door to study my data. Instead, bringing this knowledge to light has been one of the most difficult challenges of my career.

My quest to share my data with medical experts—freely and with no strings attached—began a year after my initial journey to the Ukraine. By then I had refined what I'd learned from the doctors there, and I was able to continue to supply them with new information that I had acquired with techniques developed in my own laboratories.

I was already achieving great success with human patients. I felt this was a boon for mankind that urgently needed to be shared with the medical world.

The first medical expert I approached was one of the world's first and most eminent bone marrow transplant researchers. He'd performed many successful bone marrow transplants, yet many of his initial patients had died because of graft-versus-host disease. This happened because, at the time, there was no understanding of the need for leukocyte (white blood cell) matching.

As I've said, since fetal stem cells have no antigenicity, there is no risk of graft-versus-host disease, which in turn eliminates any need for matching the donor's cells to the recipient's. I thought this discovery would be of great interest for one of the world's leading experts in bone marrow transplants, so I telephoned him and gave him a quick briefing on what I had learned.

He seemed interested, so I suggested a meeting. He agreed, and I flew to meet with him a few days later. As we talked, I felt encouraged because he clearly understood everything I was saying. I asked if he'd like to work with me to help move this important medical breakthrough along.

He looked at me. "No."

"I don't understand. Do you believe what I'm saying?"

"Yes."

"But you don't want to work with me?"

"No."

I tried a different tack: "What if you can't find a bone marrow match for a sick child? Now that you have this new information are you still are going to tell the parents of that child that he or she is going to die, even though you now know that the possibility exists that I can give you the cells to save that child's life?"

He shook his head. "I cannot work with you."

"Could you please tell me what you might be willing to do?"

He shook his head again. "No."

Because of his expertise in bone marrow transplants, this was the first doctor to fully understand the principles behind the facts I had learned. For that reason, I was desperate to get through to him. I suggested many ways by which he could address his concerns.

I suggested that he could inform his patients of my therapy without recommending it. I offered to have my attorney create a legal disclaimer stating that my treatment was experimental and that he was only informing them of it, not recommending it, thereby relieving him of any legal responsibility.

He declined.

I suggested that he could show me how to find on his computer those patients who were going to die soon for lack of a suitable bone marrow donor—and then walk out of the room. I would contact them on my own, making sure they would not have any knowledge of his involvement.

That didn't work either.

Could he put some names on a piece of paper and "accidentally" drop it on the floor? Then I'd—

"No! No! I already told you, no!"

It struck me that at that point he must be been thinking I was a complete wacko, and that I was making another enemy. So I switched to making nice, and we parted company on fairly good terms.

Another attempt was with a renowned oncologist, the chief physician and chairman of the board of one of the leading bone marrow transplant hospital in the United States. When I reached him on the phone, I introduced myself and then asked him if he knew who I was. At that time I was somewhat known because of my work on television as a medical expert; I thought it would help with my creditability if he knew of me. He did.

So I began explaining why fetal stem cell therapy would solve many problems for the bone marrow transplant process. I went through my whole monologue—no antigenicity, no matching problems, and so on.

He asked no questions but seemed to listen to everything I had to say. Then I asked, "Are you interested in joining with me to advance this research? If so, I'll come to see you at your earliest convenience."

He said, "No, I'm not interested."

Remembering my previous experience, I backpedaled and politely asked, "Would it be all right if I sent you some written material, some of my case histories, research results, or anything else you might desire?"

"No, thank you. I'm really not interested in any further conversation or information."

End of conversation.

It was mind-boggling. This eminent doctor, head of a major bone marrow transplant hospital, didn't want to even glance at any written material about a new technique that claimed to save many lives that would otherwise have been lost.

It still astounds me that these doctors, although they were sophisticated and knowledgeable enough to understand what I was telling them, would still refuse to listen,

Why? My best guess is that, due to the "political incorrectness" of using fetal stem cells; they were "covering their asses."

Another confounding episode began when I had a hypothesis about a cure for AIDS, which has since been proven correct, as you will read about later in the book.

I was able to contact the doctor who was recognized as the world's leading expert on AIDS. He agreed to see me, so I flew out east to visit him. I explained my hypothesis, backed up by my initial research, and he agreed with my assumptions. I became very excited.

"Please, work with me," I pleaded. "I just know it will work, and we can cure AIDS." I added that I was not seeking credit. I even offered to give him everything I had learned and to help him as much as I could. I explained that I had the personal resources to pay for the research, thereby eliminating any need for outside funding.

I suggested that we could bring in other researchers in his field who would want to work with us, and together, we could potentially rid the world of this terrible scourge.

For the first time, I wasn't summarily turned down.

The noted AIDS expert thanked me for sharing the exciting possibilities of this new information. He promised to think about how he could support my efforts and test my theory. He then said he would contact me to discuss a plan for going forward. I was elated. Finally, I had a heavyweight in my corner!

Two weeks later, I received a letter from him. To my surprise and dismay, it said that, with regrets, he couldn't be associated in any form or manner with the use of fetal stem cells. After giving it careful consideration, he felt the political climate was such that working with fetal stem cells could possibly result in the loss of his substantial government grants. He added that he also was unwilling to put me in touch with anyone in his field.

Why are doctors so cynical? Sadly, the American medical establishment is able to rule by fear and inertia. Doctors learn there can be negative consequences for interfering with the status quo or challenging the conventional wisdom. Therefore, the prevailing paradigm continues.

I was very disappointed by the letter, but I continued my quest.

My Quest, or Brick Walls and Deaf Ears

In the 2004 election, California had on its ballot Proposition 71, the California Stem Cell Research and Cures Initiative, which would provide $3 billion for stem cell research. I called one of the leading proponents attempting to pass the initiative. I explained to him what I had accomplished treating patients with fetal stem cells and told him I was very excited for him and for the possibility of his initiative's success.

He said that he was very impressed with what I had been able to accomplish, and that if the initiative passed he would very much like to meet in person to discuss the possibility of working together.

I took care to make sure he understood several critical points. He should not openly discuss what I had told him, since he might lose votes because of the relationship between fetal stem cells and abortion. I was financially independent and would under no circumstances accept any government funding because of the control associated with it. I was willing to share openly and freely what I had learned over the past 10 years and wanted nothing in return other than the information being placed in the public realm, thus moving stem cell research ahead 20 years. He expressed gratitude for my "very generous offer."

The bill passed and we set up an appointment at my office the following week. When we met, we spontaneously hugged each other in excitement. I congratulated him and his fellow supporters who had worked so hard on its success and then warned that, in my experience, the actual funds would be a long time coming due to the powerful forces acting against embryonic stem cell research.

That is indeed what happened. The California Institute for Regenerative Medicine (CIRM), the organization that would receive the

75

$3 billion and use it to fund the research, quickly became tied up in litigation. I was told at one point they were actually sued by an *embryo.*

A member of the board of CIRM knew of the parents of one of my patients, who had been told by their doctor that, due to excessive brain damage, their son had only a few months to live…and also knew that, thanks to fetal stem cell therapy, that child was alive and doing well four years later.

We made the following plans: When CIRM was close to receiving the funds, which would be made available at the rate of $300 million a year for 10 years; arrangements would be made for me to freely disseminate all my research in an open forum of scientists and board members for evaluation and possible acceptance as a template for CIRM's future research.

A short while later, the medical director of CIRM issued a press release which included his belief that, in ten years, after all the allocated $3 billion was spent, they might possibly have a treatment for one illness. I was surprised and found it strange that the medical director was either unaware or unwilling to discuss the research plan that we had decided on.

After CIRM first began to receive funding, I read in *the Los Angeles Times that they were about to allocate over $200 million to build research buildings and to train new mouse researchers.* I immediately called CIRM and offered to meet in the San Francisco office. I was called back, and we set a time to meet. This appointment as well as two others was then cancelled on short notice. Subsequent calls to the office went unanswered.

During this time, I continued to read newspaper stories of how more and more of California's government money was being spent on erecting buildings and training new mouse researchers.

I was finally able to reach a CIRM board member and explained to him that if I were ever to be asked if CIRM in any way was aware of my research as well as my willingness to freely share it, I would tell the truth. I did not want to now or ever in the future receive a grant. I simply wanted their scientific panel to evaluate my results and then have more information when making their decision as to the future research direction of CIRM.

I told him the public would then know that in a struggling California economy, CIRM had spent billions of dollars on years of mouse research while completely ignoring my human data. He said he understood and would call me back. The call never came.

The following are public statements from The California Institute of Regenerative Medicine:

Helping to educate and inform the next generation of scientists is an important part of CIRM's outreach mission.

The California Institute of Regenerative Medicine has already awarded $761 million in research and facilities grants—and has brought in roughly one billion dollars more additional funding in matching grants and donations. An incredible 300 published scientific papers resulting from CIRM-funded work brings us incrementally closer to cures for chronic disease and disability.[xiii]

Nearly 2 billion dollars—and the many thousands of research hours involved in generating 300 research papers—all to bring us "incrementally closer" to treatments and cures? What an unconscionable waste of resources! This money could be spent treating patients instead of funding hundreds of researchers' careers for the next 20 years.

One of the definitions of medical malpractice is the use of a treatment that falls outside of the standard of medical care. That is, doing something different from what the other doctors do in the same set of clinical circumstances. Unfortunately, it appears this attitude has carried over from clinical practice into the world of research.

"Medical correctness" can create an environment of fear that interferes with the spirit of adventure and intellectual curiosity, which may eventually lead to great medical breakthroughs.

A Doctor Who Believed

Never doubt that a small group of thoughtful, committed citizens can change the world. Indeed, it is the only thing that ever has.

—Margret Meade

Despite all the people who have refused to consider and study my work, there was one eminent American doctor who became a believer in fetal stem cell therapy—by virtue of being a patient.

This case history just might finally convince physicians to sit up and take notice. Why? Because it's told by one of their own, a prominent surgeon.

Dr. Dennis Nigro's life as a doctor was rich and meaningful. A former college athlete and hard-core yoga and exercise fanatic, he was in fantastic physical shape. But in just one heartbeat, Dr. Nigro's life was shattered the day he received a frightening diagnosis of a deadly disease.

Dr. Nigro was told he had—at best—two months to live. He would soon become my patient.

One evening I received a phone call from Brian Novak, an internationally renowned plastic surgeon and close friend.

He said, "Hi, Bill, hope I'm not interrupting dinner, but I've got a colleague who really needs your help."

"You're not interrupting anything, Brian. What's up?"

"Bill, I'm calling about a Dr. Dennis Nigro. You may have heard of him. He's the Chief of Plastic Surgery at Scripps Memorial Hospital in San Diego. He's the fellow who founded Fresh Start years ago, that charity group of surgeons that gives free craniofacial surgery to deformed children. Dennis flies all around the world helping these poor kids.

"He's one of those guys who work out like Schwarzenegger, an outstanding athlete at Notre Dame, lifting weights and actually doing about a thousand sit-ups a day. But the other day, right out of the blue, Dennis was in the middle of operating on a patient when he suddenly became woozy. They rushed him to the emergency room. Four days later, he got the diagnosis—stage four cancer of the esophagus and it's already spread to the liver. He has only a few months, at best. He tells me he's scheduled to start chemotherapy tomorrow. I told him what you've done with the fetal stem cells, and said he just had to talk to you first. Bill, can you help him?"

"I believe I can but he has to call me immediately, tonight."

"Done."

"Now here comes the hard part, Brian. He's got to take my advice on a treatment plan, and there will be no real time to think it over. He's got to take action tomorrow morning. Will that be a problem? He doesn't know me or my work, right?"

"Bill, I told him about your research and your incredible track record. Dr. Nigro's a really smart guy, one of the best in his field. And he knows a lot about the immune system. He helped edit a textbook on it when he was in med school. Tell him your plan. I believe he'll listen."

Ten minutes after I hung up the phone, it rang again. It was Dr. Nigro. I listened very closely to his story. From his reactions to my comments, I knew almost instantly that I was going to be his doctor. What he told me was unforgettable.

I've asked him to tell his entire story in his own words for this book.

My scrub nurse was just handing me what I needed to make the final suture on my facial reconstruction patient when the lights in the operating room suddenly seemed to flicker.

I began feeling weak, woozy. It was that sensation I remember from being slammed in football games, when you see stars and flashing lights. Holding on to the operating table, I dropped my head below my shoulders to regain my equilibrium. My OR clinical staff looked startled. When I spontaneously started to sweat profusely, they made me lie down and hooked me up to monitors. Somebody said, "Is he having a heart attack?"

I answered, "No way!"

But nobody was listening to the doctor now.

My staff called 911. An ambulance rushed me across the street to the emergency room at Scripps Memorial Hospital Encinitas.

The staff there all knows me. I'm Chief of Plastic Surgery. They went all-out, examining me urgently, conducting tests, trying to figure out what the heck was wrong with this guy they knew as the picture of perfect health. It was an incredibly surreal moment.

The day had started like any other. I woke at 4 a.m., put on a 60-pound weight vest, clipped 15-pound weights on each ankle, and exercised for about 45 minutes on my elliptical trainer.

I followed that with about 1,000 stomach exercises on various machines, then did about 200 reps of arm, shoulder, and back exercises, using 35-pound dumbbells. Then, at 6:30 a.m., I headed off for a yoga class.

Sounds a little extreme, doesn't it?

I'm not mentioning all this to brag. I'm just pointing out that my lifestyle is so healthy that people often kid me about it. I'm very compulsive about my diet and supplements. I take regular blood tests. In other words, there was no reason for this episode, unless it was caused by something like not drinking enough water that day.

Initial lab studies in the emergency room came back normal, except for a slight drop in my hemoglobin count. Testing for blood in my GI tract and urine was negative. The emergency room doctor suggested I stay overnight for follow-ups. I declined. I felt fine, now that I'd been given some fluids; it was all very puzzling. But I'm a doctor, so I did my own follow-ups.

I had no patients until 10 the next morning, so at 8 a.m., Dr. Philip Kumar, a gastroenterologist, kindly changed his schedule and gave me an endoscopy, looking into my stomach with a lighted instrument.

He did a number of biopsies, but didn't see anything except a small irregularity in one area. There was no gross bleeding or suggestion of an ulcer. I examined the pictures of my stomach. Tissues would be available for examination next day.

My medical assistant, Lisa Parker, was driving me back to my office, when I involuntarily blurted, "I think this might be cancer."

I couldn't believe what I'd said. It had just popped out. Lisa was shaken. So was I.

Back at the office, I kept it business-as-usual and saw patients. But I couldn't shake off the lurking premonition. And I couldn't figure out why.

My wife Brenda had been on vacation in Utah with my two daughters, Bergen, who was eight, and Erris, four. They came home immediately.

The next day I spoke to a pathologist who'd examined the slides of my tissues. He told me, "Don't worry about it, Dennis. It's just an inflammation. I don't see much there." Brenda and I, naturally on pins and needles, breathed a sigh of relief. It was miraculous that I'd been spared, I thought.

Then...trouble.

Over the next 36 hours, my blood count began to drop dangerously. I lost about one third of my blood volume. I needed to be transfused. Then the initial biopsy reports came back. They indicated "benign or inflammatory fibrosis." I ordered a CAT scan on myself, then stayed overnight in the hospital and received three units of blood. The next morning I phoned my friend Dr. Brunst, the expert who'd read my CAT scan, with my wife listening in. I immediately knew by his distraught tone that he had bad news.

He told me, "Dennis, you have stage four cancer of the lower esophagus, with metastases—a lot of them—to your liver and lymph nodes."

Brenda broke down and sobbed. I was shocked. Oddly enough, I felt no despair for myself at that moment, but I was devastated by the effect the news had on my wife. Brenda was inconsolable. A fog descended, permeating everything. Facing the possibility that my life would end within months, we tried desperately to think of what we needed to do. I'm a doctor, so naturally I started seeking opinions from cancer centers around the country, and from our own UCSD Cancer Center.

The feedback was dismal. It looked like there was no magic bullet out there for me. I was only prolonging the inevitable. I knew what it would be like, and I was terrified.

In the short term, we needed to slow down my internal bleeding. I took treatments in a hyperbaric chamber, crawling inside a closed steel cylinder saturated with high-pressure oxygen. The bleeding abated, but my hours inside that chamber were lonely and scary. I felt totally isolated. There was nothing to do but think about the fate that awaited me. I thought about how I would miss the joy of watching my little girls grow up. I had such dreams for their lives! On my first day in the hyperbaric chamber, I wrote them a letter.

July 13, 2008

Dearest Bergen and Erris,

I'm sitting in a giant metal tube which pumps large amounts of life-giving oxygen into me in the hopes that it will help me, as I'm pretty sick. I thought I would write down some thoughts to share with you, and that you can have in the future.

I have always made a point to tell you that I love you both more than words can tell every day. Every day, I have hugged you and told you that I love you, but my words could not possibly give a fair idea of what that really means. I'm not sure I really know, except that there is no greater yearning for connection I have ever known.

I wish I could explain this better, but one day, the first day one of your babies is born, you will know. I want you to know that my love is eternal and unconditional, and if for some reason in the future you don't hear that, know it is being said over and over. Listen to your heart; the sound it makes is your mommy and I telling you we love you, and we will always be with you.

My Eternal Love,
Daddy

At a certain point, after a continuous barrage of dismal information about my condition, my family and I came to the conclusion that there was nothing left to do but play out the last few months of my life. Strangely, I just didn't feel that it was "my time." I had so many missions in life. But in 36 hours, my hopes and dreams for my family and myself had been turned upside down. And I couldn't help but worry about what would happen to the charitable craniofacial clinic for children that I'd started 20 years ago.

I've never considered myself a person of great faith, but I try to be a faithful person. As a child, I attended Catholic school, became an altar boy, and tried to speak to God.

I went to a Jesuit prep school, then to Notre Dame, and on to a Catholic medical school. I'd lived a faith-based life. Now I needed a lifeline to God, in the truest sense of the word. After all my science and study, what I needed was a miracle.

Friends rallied around me, especially those from Notre Dame, where I'd been the third generation in my family to graduate. I got phone calls from Notre Dame athletic coaches, including the great Lou Holtz.

Many members of the alumni association called, and we prayed together. I admit it seemed like it would be all for naught, but their faith never wavered.

On my way into work one morning, a good friend and patient of mine who lived in Paris texted me to say she'd be passing through Los Angeles and wanted to visit us. I know her well, so I texted back and disclosed my medical problems. She was shocked.

She immediately contacted a fellow plastic surgeon, Dr. Brian Novak, who called me and said, "Don't you dare do anything until I put you in touch with my friend and colleague, Dr. William Rader."

Dr. Novak brought me up to speed on Dr. Rader's work and recommended him highly. I called Dr. Rader and he said: "Dr. Novak talked to me about your condition. Listen, you are going to be fine. We can beat this with a regimen that will utilize fetal stem cells to not only attack the cancer but also to allow you to tolerate chemoembolization of the affected areas and begin to gain control of your cancer. Then I'll send you to a clinic in Europe. Radiotherapy, toxic chemotherapy and surgical intervention are not in your immediate future."

Dr. Rader seemed very knowledgeable about the concept that normally the cancer areas could not be aggressively treated. Because it also destroys the immune system, sometimes the body cannot withstand chemotherapy and survive. He made an astute analogy: The fetal stem cells, he said, would quickly give me a new immune system ten times stronger than a normal healthy adult's. This would allow me to be able to withstand even stronger doses of chemotherapy, thereby providing maximum treatment. At the same time, the fetal stem cells would also be providing rehab for the treated areas.

It made great sense to me, as a surgeon. My spirits soared. I didn't know Dr. Rader personally, but his kindred spirit galvanized me in a heartbeat. I felt as though we were on the same page psychologically. And because I have a relatively long history of understanding immunology—I helped write and edit a textbook on the subject with my professor of pathology in medical school.

I realized that his analogy was very similar to the treatment of infections. Using fetal stem cells to help rejuvenate and revitalize the structure of the cancer that had been treated was a concept that I grasped immediately.

He told me, "You know boxing, right? If I hit you in the face once, you'll dance away and try to shake it off. And if I'm dumb enough to let you do that, you'll be able to take a lot of punches. But if I hit you in the face, then quickly hit you again, and again, and again—never giving you a chance to recover—you're going to be defeated quickly. That's how it is with these cancer cells. If we hit them hard with a strong dose of chemo-therapy, it will hurt them. But under normal circumstances, if we were to immediately follow up with another strong dose, it could end up also destroying your immune system because it's too toxic. So ordinarily we have to wait between the doses of chemotherapy. But that gives the cancer time to recover and grow strong again. Fetal stem cell therapy will let us keep hitting that cancer hard and fast until it's down for the count and at the same time revitalize your devastated areas."

Dr. Rader paused, and then said, "I can tell what kind of doctor you are. I'm the same. Put your trust in me. I believe I can save your life.

First, you must cancel the chemotherapy that's been scheduled for tomorrow."

I know it sounds unbelievable and a bit crazy, but Dr. Rader's professionalism and confidence buoyed me with such hope that Brenda and I immediately launched preparations for a trip to his clinic for me to receive fetal stem cells. We had to be there in 36 hours, and then immediately thereafter go on to the clinic he recommended in Munich, Germany. The journey I was about to take with Dr. Rader was launched with hope and fear, but somehow I felt God's will had directed me onto this path.

Within a few days, we arrived at Dr. Rader's clinic. The fetal stem cell therapy was administered at his direction.

Procedure

It was very quick and painless. Hematopoietic (blood) cells were injected intravenously, and neuronal (nerve) cells were delivered subcutaneously, through little needle-pricks under the skin.

My first reaction after receiving the fetal stem cells was that I felt incredibly invigorated.

"There's no time to waste," said Dr. Rader after the procedure. "It's off to Germany."

As we rushed off by car and then boarded the plane, I was already feeling relief from the ever-present aches and pains caused by old orthopedic injuries—and I have many, including six knee operations from football injuries, a shoulder dislocation, and broken thumbs. By the time we arrived at the airport in Munich, I felt like I didn't need a taxi into the city; I could've run the distance! That's how good I felt already.

When we arrived at the clinic, we were met by Dr. Ursula Jacob, who had my entire treatment plan ready. Extensive tests that would've taken weeks to get approved in the United States were conducted immediately. Two days later I had my first appointment with Dr. Thomas Vogl, a world-renowned interventional radiologist at Goethe University.

Dr. Vogl explained that he was going to put a catheter in my groin, run it up into my liver, and begin a series of chemoembolization of my tumors—injecting toxic chemotherapy right into them. He knew that because I'm a doctor myself I would understand a lot of this, so his descriptions were quite detailed. Then, under local anesthesia, I actually got to witness the entire procedure on the screen of a gigantic 3-D CT scanner. I watched as the catheter was threaded up my femoral artery and climbed up my aorta. I could feel it bumping into the inside of my liver. And when Dr. Vogel sprayed the affected area internally with a liquid that showed up on the arteriogram, I actually felt it bathing my insides, like warm water. Finally, Dr. Vogl and I watched the chemotherapy agents being introduced into my cancerous tumors.

"Well, we'll see—it should be fine," Dr. Vogl said. Then he rolled me into the waiting room. I was there about four hours. Then Brenda drove us the five hours back to Munich. All during the trip I was careful not to let on that I was filled with dread.

Why? I didn't tell her, but I had actually seen my arteriogram.

It looked, in a word, terrible. There were tumors all over my liver. They were vascular and they appeared to be highly aggressive. Fortunately, they were still in the peripheral liver.

They had not gotten deep into the substance or near important ducts, although there was one that was quite close. The doctors had gone inside in the nick of time. But would the treatment be successful? It was too early to tell. I knew I had to hang tough.

In the days that followed, a routine began.

I would arrive at the Munich clinic by 6 a.m. An hour later, Dr. Vogl would begin treating my liver with supportive things like vitamin therapy and homeopathic agents.

But my ace in the hole was Dr. Rader's fetal stem cells. They were protecting my immune system and servicing my damaged areas, repairing them quickly so that I could have more chemotherapy.

A couple of days after my initial treatment, Dr. Jacob began ultrasound examinations. To my absolute astonishment, they clearly showed that the metastases on my liver had undergone great change. They looked like they were dying. In just four days, the change to the right lobe of my liver was flat-out amazing—shocking, actually. I was filled with sudden hope as I watched those terrifying tumors dematerialize. Even Dr. Jacob and Dr. Vogl were surprised. Dr. Vogl had originally told me that we'd only be able to initiate chemotherapy once every three weeks because it was so incredibly toxic.

But now Dr. Rader's prophecy began to come true.

"Dennis, your liver will respond just fine," he'd told me. "You'll be able to continue aggressive treatment and get this under control fast."

And that's exactly what happened. My liver enzymes stayed rock solid. As a result, I could receive the chemotherapy once a week for four weeks. Dr. Vogl, who has treated thousands of patients, said he'd never seen such a response. All the tumors shrunk in those four weeks, and my primary tumor had decreased to about 30 percent of its original size. After my final chemoembolization therapy, Brenda and I flew back to San Diego.

I went back to work, albeit minimally, just four days later. I underwent tests and showed no serious side effects from the treatments. This was amazing, considering the amount of poison that had been injected and how quickly my tissues had healed. The fetal stem cells had protected me.

I pressed on and even began my exercise regimen again, although I'm not nearly as physically fit as I had been.

Make no mistake. This is still a fight—with no whistle, no clock, and no time-outs. The struggle begins again every morning. There's no flinching or backing off.

But being alive when you were told you would be dead is a miraculous thing. I simply put my trust in God's hands and Dr. Rader's unwavering confidence in fetal stem cell therapy.

Today, as I—cancer patient, doctor, observer, scientist, child of God—struggle and fight, I know I've been given a great blessing. When I underwent those treatments and watched those scanners, I struck a lot of deals with God. But as I passed each diagnostic test, I felt a halo encircling me.

And I promised that I would be the messenger—the one who would tell the world about this wonderful gift of nature that is healing me, these fetal stem cells.

One of my favorite passages in the Bible commands: "From those who have been given much, much is required" (Luke, 12:48).

Today we sit astride a monumental opportunity. But we must not sit idly. How many more souls must suffer? How many babies, children, and adults will face agony and even death because the benefits of fetal stem cells go uninvestigated, their potential untapped? Not so long ago, we thought the world was flat. That's what the evidence of our eyes showed us. But have we not yet learned that there's much that doesn't meet the eye?

Step forward with me, and help unlock what might be the greatest medical miracle of our time. Help Dr. Rader in his quest to unleash the potential of this therapy from the future that promises to bring hope, health, and happiness to countless generations.

I am a physician, and I believe in the fetal stem cell miracle. I have lived it, participated in its marvels. Its time has come. Stories like mine do not occur by chance. What happened is a message. Heed it. Please.

It grieves me to report that more than a year after being told he had at most just two months to live, Dr. Dennis Nigro suddenly died following unexpected consequences from an oncological surgical procedure here in the United States. The world has lost a man of great mind, character and heart. And even though some critics may cite his death as a failure of fetal stem cell therapy, I have included his story because – as you know from reading his own words – Dr. Nigro was passionate about the soundness and potential of the science that he had observed, and he wanted the truth to be told.

His wife, Brenda not only approved the inclusion of his story, she wrote this note for me to share with you:

Dear Dr. Rader,

My husband passed away almost a year to the day after he wrote those touching, treasured letters of love and hope to our daughters you've included in your book. Anyone reading what Dennis wrote as he sat alone in that hyperbaric chamber can sense his apprehension that time was running out very quickly indeed.

What happened next was a miracle. Your swift intervention with fetal stem cell therapy gave us a fighting chance. Suddenly, my husband was healing! Despite his ordeal and the knowledge that he wasn't out of the woods yet, my daughters and I had many months of joy and love with our husband and father.

But Dennis was a doctor, after all, and knew he was fighting a malignant killer. And finally, after undergoing a medical procedure, Dennis was gone.

Bill, my husband wanted so passionately for you to continue the pioneering work you've started. Please, with all my heart and his spirit, I urge you: Do not falter. The world needs the stem cell miracle.

Sincerely,
Brenda Nigro

Lies, Myths, Misconceptions, and Mice

You can count the seeds in an apple, but you can't count the apples in a seed.

—Proverb

One of the reasons fetal stem cell therapy has yet to enter the mainstream of scientific research is the widespread attacks on its validity—criticisms that are erroneous and, in many cases, self-serving to the critics.

The road to realizing the medical benefits of this therapy is blocked by the confluence of political, economic, and socio-religious factors driven by vested interests, misguided beliefs, and ignorance. The synergy of these forces has kept fetal stem cell treatment from becoming widely available for those who need it most. Were this not the case, health care as we know it today could significantly change almost overnight.

The most pernicious lie is the often-repeated contention that not one human being has ever been helped by fetal stem cells. This falsehood has been widely disseminated by the religious right, pharmaceutical companies, politicians, and even the media.

One of the most frustrating sources of denial has been those in the best position to evaluate the results of fetal stem cell therapy—the personal physicians themselves. Typically, my patients return to their doctors bursting with joyful news of their successful outcomes. Too often the very same doctors who told them that their case was hopeless ignore the evidence in front of their eyes and often suggest that these patients are deluded by their fervent hope for recovery.

I find it hard to forgive physicians who consistently ignore the evidence before them: patients who have experienced dramatic improvements or even full recoveries from their "hopeless" conditions. Apparently doctors, like anybody else, can be reluctant to accept something that might turn their previous knowledge and experience upside down.

The publication of this book will, I believe, put pressure on the gatekeepers of science to publish my professional data and treat it fairly. Until that happens, cynical doctors will, no doubt, continue to disbelieve my "deluded" patients.

Perhaps you know the story of the blind men and the elephant. Six learned blind men go to observe an elephant to learn what that creature is like. Each man touches but one part of the elephant, and in turn they pronounce the beast to be exactly like a wall, a fan, a tree, a spear, a rope, or a snake.

The primary physician of a patient who has received fetal stem cell therapy is like those blind men. Typically, he has never encountered any other such case, and so more often than not, he writes off the miraculous results with the meaningless phrase: "You have had a spontaneous recovery"

I am a doctor fortunate enough to have seen the whole elephant. I have treated more than 1,500 patients with fetal stem cells. I want to share my research data so that everyone can recognize the elephant for what it really is. Moreover, in each of these cases, there is someone who is in a better position than anyone else, including myself, to judge the treatment's outcome: the patient, or the parent of the patient.

It is extremely difficult to shatter the paradigms and conventional wisdom of the current medical establishment. Many of what the FDA, scientists, and researchers hold to be established medical truths have, throughout history, turned out to be wrong.

A recent example is the old saying about taking it easy on your alcohol consumption because "as an adult, you can never get back those lost brain cells." In 1999, scientists discovered for the first time that you actually do continue to grow new brain cells, albeit a limited number, throughout your adult life. (As a doctor who has done a great deal of work in the field of alcoholism and addiction treatment, I must add that this obviously should not be interpreted in any way as a rationale for excessive drinking).

Here's another erroneous statement still accepted as scientific gospel: stem cells cannot cross the blood-brain barrier. Many of the case histories of my patients prove irrefutably that fetal stem cells can indeed cross the blood-brain barrier: a blind, brain-damaged child who can now see, an Alzheimer's patient whose mind is now clear, as well as innumerable other examples.

For example, some of my patients' brain scans show actual brain cortex growth after a traumatic brain injury; MRIs of others more often than not indicate that the plaques in the brain from multiple sclerosis have disappeared.

Relatively unknown case studies in the medical literature not only validate my findings but also prove that the "experts" can be completely wrong. One class of such cases involved women who received bone marrow transplants from male donors. Researchers examined post mortem samples from female patients who had received bone marrow transplants from male donors. They found that many of the subjects had numerous brain cells containing the Y-chromosome, which could have come only from the male donors cells crossing the blood brain barrier.

The U.S. National Institute of Neurological Diseases and Stroke research team concluded that immature cells from the bone marrow traveled to the subjects' brains and became fully functioning brain cells, adding that their findings "could eventually inspire novel treatments for brain trauma and diseases such as Alzheimer's and Parkinson's."[xiv]

New scientific developments like this one are a time bomb for the pharmaceutical industry. Fetal stem cell treatment that can cross the blood brain barrier could render obsolete many of their drugs, both current and in development, thereby costing these companies billions of dollars in sales.

But their loss will be an equivalent gain for humanity—including consumers, taxpayers, and patients.

Today, pharmaceutical companies work in collusion with the FDA, the National Institutes of Health (NIH) and universities and institutions by awarding them millions of dollars in research grants. Many such grants would be revoked if fetal stem cells were allowed to take their deserved position in modern-day medicine.

In 2001, well-known university researcher Dr. James Thomson was on the cover of *Time magazine* as "the man who brought you stem cells." Dr. Thomson is credited with having derived the first human embryonic stem cell line. It had been announced that Dr. Thomson would begin the first mouse studies in the near future, with human use predicted to be 20 years away. At the time that article was published, *I had already been administering fetal stem cell therapy to human patients for more than five years.*

I am not the only doctor or scientist to bemoan the influence that the pharmaceutical industry exerts over doctors and the integrity of scientific research. Reuters recently cited prominent medical educators criticizing conflicts of interest, such as the many perks doctors receive from drug companies. The Reuters article quoted Dr. Harlan Krumholz of Yale University: "We've seen a lot of transgressions—people will take advantage of the system for their own self-aggrandizement or profit. It's got to stop."

Dr. Marsha Angell of Harvard Medical School, a former editor of the New England Journal of Medicine, said that "there should be no relationship between the drug industry and either prescribers or patients." She argued that doctors should pay for their own continuing medical education rather than rely on updates from drug companies on their own products. She added that doctors' professional organizations should not ask drug companies to subsidize the cost of meetings and publications. "You might have to go down to the local high school instead of playing golf in Hawaii, but the education would be better because it would be impartial," Angell said.

Finally, Washington health policy analyst Scott Gottlieb told Reuters that drug makers should focus more on advancing science than on marketing.[xv]

Thanks to the change of occupants in the White House, expanded stem cell research is now possible, and the tide of public

By William C. Rader, MD

opinion is swiftly turning in its favor. If this seems like great news, I am sorry to burst your bubble. In all probability, all that new research money will be allocated to scientists conducting more studies on mice.

A recent discovery in stem cell research—induced pluripotent stem cells— has garnered a great deal of attention. Induced pluripotent stem cells (IPSC) are derived from skin cells. They supposedly have properties similar to those of embryonic stem cells. Receiving less than adequate attention is the fact that in order to create these cells, two retroviruses and two genes must be added. One of the retroviruses and one of the genes can cause cancer. Researchers say this problem can be solved sometime in the future.

According to an article dated May 2009, from The Scripps Research Institute and others, regarding the creation of induced pluripotent stem cells:

All of the methods developed to date still involve the use of genetic materials and thus the potential for unexpected genetic modifications.

A Stanford Office of Technology Article:

Stanford researchers have identified a way in which teratomas (a cancer that contains hair, skin, bone and teeth), can be detected. According to the researchers: Teratoma formation is a potentially severe complication of using cellular derivatives, such as **induced pluripotent stem cells (iPS)**, *in clinical treatment.*

Another futile waste of time, effort, and a great deal of money is stem cell researchers' dealing with the problem of rejection *(which is nonexistent using fetal stem cells).* They remove the nucleus from a patient's own cell and insert it into a donor egg that has had its nucleus removed. This is called a somatic nuclear transplant.

A South Korean doctor made headlines when he declared that he had succeeded in this process. He made more headlines when it was discovered he had faked his results. However, the technique is still being studied as a way of preventing rejection, or graft-versus-host disease. Yet the whole question should be moot. By now you have learned why: Since fetal stem cells have no antigenicity, rejection is not an issue.

Another advantage of fetal stem cell therapy that is denied by the medical establishment is the way in which fetal stem cells help compensate for the patient's own genetic flaws. I'll explain this by analogy. If I were to ask you what type of dog is the healthiest, smartest, and best adjusted, you would probably choose a particular breed. In fact, the answer is a mutt—a dog containing genetic material from multiple sources. As you may be aware, purebred dogs often have genetic defects, most commonly hip dysplasia. Similarly, so do the descendents of "purebred" humans, such as royalty (the most common affliction being epilepsy).

Although they retain their own genetic make-up, after receiving fetal stem cells, patients become mutts in a sense, with all the associated benefits thereof—including a new strong, healthy immune system.

If fetal stem cell treatment were to become readily available, as I believe it eventually will, medicine would change dramatically and health care would be much more efficient and effective. There would also be huge benefits with regard to perhaps the greatest political and economic issue in America today: reducing our ballooning health care costs.

Or we can continue to ignore and deny the benefits of fetal stem cells and continue to endure the burden of unnecessary suffering, premature death, and exploding costs.

Success Stories: Making the Case for Fetal Stem Cell Therapy

Search for the cure within the cause. The body itself is the best physician.

—Plato

Stem cell therapy is the first area of medicine that's not primarily based on drugs. It is nature's medicine, not man's pharmacological chemistry set.

—William C. Rader, MD

Having treated more than 1,500 patients, I cannot present all my case histories in a single book, but I will introduce many so-called "hopeless" patients most representative of the impact that fetal stem cells can make. These stories encompass a wide range of diseases and disorders. You will also read riveting accounts of how fetal stem cell therapy can help reverse the effects of human aging, increase longevity, and enhance one's overall quality of life.

The fetal stem cell miracle is already with us. I hope that after you have read these case histories of my patients, you will agree that each one stands as evidence sufficient to warrant launching full-scale research into fetal stem cell therapy.

Think about it. If I, with very limited financial resources, was able to achieve this degree of success, imagine what could be accomplished with the billions of dollars, primarily funded through our tax dollars, allocated each year for medical research in the United States.

Imagine what thousands of well-funded physicians, scientists, and researchers— starting with what I have learned over the past 15 years— could create for the future of medicine and the benefit of mankind.

Wherever possible, I have presented my patients' case histories in their own words, gleaned from the actual letters and e-mails they and their families were kind enough to send us for our follow-up studies. These patients' stories clearly illustrate the power of fetal stem cells to effect repair and recovery. To protect the privacy of my patients, I have changed their names. Of course, some of my patients have not received the same level of benefit as the ones whose stories I have included. But as a group, they have exhibited healing and recovery well beyond any other medical intervention they had previously undergone.

They have told their stories with an honesty and eloquence that bespeaks truth. If these stories move you as they have me, I hope you will help advance the case for fetal stem cell therapy by sharing them with your physician.

In Their Own Words

In the preceding chapters I have made my own arguments on behalf of fetal stem therapy. I have discussed the validity of the treatment, the science behind it, and the political and cultural opposition I have faced.

Now it is time to hear from those who can argue this case most compellingly: the people who have benefited from fetal stem cell therapy.

I'll start by sharing just a few of the letters I have received.

I am presenting them in their entirety, in their own words, including at times some kind words for me, so you can evaluate their experiences and their belief in fetal stem cell therapy. NOTE: Even though the patients' names have been changed to protect their privacy, they are real people who stand ready to meet and freely share their experiences with accredited medical experts, researchers, journalists and any others who will objectively evaluate their results from fetal stem cell treatment.

My objective is to bring fetal stem cell therapy into the mainstream of medical practice, so that the outcomes experienced by my 1,500 patients can be extended to the millions needing this treatment.

By William C. Rader, MD

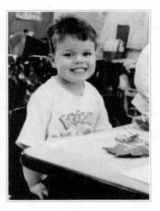

Jake before his stroke

Dear Dr. Rader,

I am sending you a summary of Jake's story, including pictures.

My son Jake suffered a series of debilitating strokes following a rare brain infection in December 2003 at the age of 5, which left him in a comatose state, severely brain damaged. After all the doctors, including the specialists, ran their many tests, they told us to discontinue any supportive medical treatment for Jake and "pull the plug."

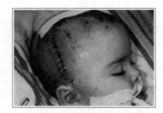

After neurosurgery

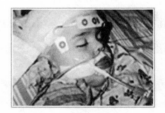

Comatose

Hearing this, we had a priest from our local parish perform the sacrament of Confirmation for Jake in lieu of last rites, since he was not old enough for original sin.

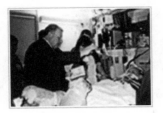

Receiving last rites

But, going against medical advice, we refused to take our son off life support.

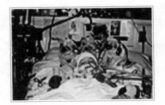

On life support

To the surprise of all his doctors, Jake slowly began to improve into what is called a minimally responsive, semi-vegetative state. He was breathing through a tracheotomy tube and being fed liquids through a "g-tube" placed in his stomach. Although he was improving, eventually Jake was left blind, unable to speak, could only minimally move his right side, and appeared to be extremely cognitively impaired.

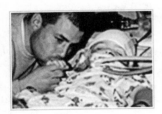
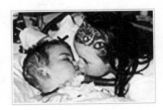

With me   With his sister

By William C. Rader, MD

This continued for three years, until I found Dr. Rader, who agreed to treat Jake with fetal stem cells. Sixty days following his first treatment, miraculously Jake began to speak, initially just a few words. Then within only a few more weeks, he had progressed to over 500 words.

Slowly but surely, Jake's speech continues to improve. He is now initiating, as well as carrying on, conversations with us and others. Now his vision is starting to return. His left side, which was completely paralyzed, has begun to move...his much-improved right side and all of his extremities are becoming much stronger. His tracheotomy has been removed, because he breathes normally, and he is now able to feed himself.

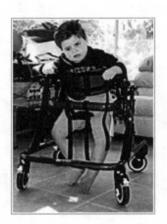

Four months after the Fetal Stem Cells

The progress we see in Jake continues to build every day with no regression.

My son Jake calls the fetal stem cells "miracle juice."

They say the creation of life is miraculous. Well, then maybe Jake is right; they should be called miracle juice. I know that's what they are in our house.

I firmly believe that the fetal stem cells have dramatically improved my son's level of function. My family feels they have transformed my son's life, giving our family hope and giving Jake a quality of life we were assured would be impossible for him to achieve.

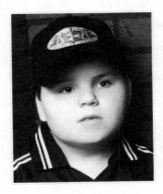

Jake today

Dear Dr. Rader,

The following is an update of my medical history:

My initial debilitating medical problem was diagnosed over two and a half years ago as severe peripheral neuropathy, as a result of an artificial disk that was placed in my spine at the L-5, S-1 location, because of my chronic mild-to-moderate back pain.

The damage almost certainly evolved from the lead surgeon severely overstretching my spinal cord during a surgery that lasted over nine hours. When I got up the next day after the surgery, I had excruciating pain from the waist down, and no feeling in my feet and part of my right leg, something I had never felt before in my entire life. I have not been right since.

My doctor assured me that in time everything would become normal again. I kept my trust in his word. Over the next six months I kept insisting to him that something was really wrong with my legs and feet. However, it kept falling on deaf ears. All he wanted was to talk about was my back pain. I told him, very well, but I was much more concerned about my other frightening symptoms, which he was refusing to deal with or really even acknowledge.

Since I could not get him to listen, I went to another doctor, who performed a nerve conductive study. The results were that I had severe peripheral neuropathy in both legs and feet, from the knees to the ends of my feet. This doctor too had nothing to offer me.

As someone who is not prone to exaggeration, to try to explain to you the level of my unbearable pain, it actually felt as if a 10-ton road compactor had rolled over and crushed both of my feet flat as a pancake and then lit them on fire...the bottoms of my feet felt as if someone had sewn small jagged lumps of coal in them. My calf muscles were also in excruciating pain, as if I had torn every ligament, tendon, and muscle in each of them, with the right leg being even worse than the left.

When I would try to walk up stairs I just did not have the muscle strength needed to do it. I had to use my arms to pull myself up by the railings. I lived in constant hell, with all that pain, and no matter what I tried, I was unable to get any relief from the nightmare that I was living in.

I finally went to another doctor who thought maybe a wheelchair, crutches, or a walker might help in my daily activities. My response was that this was not an option, that I had not, nor would I ever give in to this condition, and that I must find a cure. It was at that time he explained to me that I was disabled and that he would issue me a handicapped sticker so that I wouldn't have to walk as far. Again I explained to him that I was not handicapped and would continue to search for a cure that he assured me did not exist.

Another year went by with me continuing to try every possibility for any type of relief that I was able to find, including laser treatment, TENS (transcutaneous electrical nerve stimulation) treatment, EMS (electromagnetic stimulation) treatments, and many more. Again, nothing worked.

I was mentally exhausted, I could hardly think straight, and I was alienating everyone around me because of a very short temper. All of this because I was in severe, unrelenting pain from the moment I woke up until the time I finally went to bed.

Which leads me to about 3 months ago. I decided I had not been back to my original doctor in over a year, so I went back to him again, thinking maybe there would be some new magic bullet, and instead here were the options that were given to me: Either get a portable pump so that I could press a button and inject morphine into my veins, or have a device surgically implanted into me permanently that would dispense the morphine automatically. Either of these options would have assured I would end up as a hardcore morphine addict. A third and final option was to just continue to live in agony. Pardon me, but I let him know in harsh terms that none of the suggestions were in any way acceptable to me.

I brought up the possibility that stem cells might be of some help to me. He immediately told me that there was not any proof that could work, that I was not being realistic and was just wasting my time.

He then said, "You are a very hard-headed man, and you do not get that you are at a dead end." I told him I was going to search the entire world until I found a cure and when that happened I would come back to him with new muscles and a new attitude and that I would not be denied.

When I went back to my car from his office, I cried for the first time in many years. My daughter called me later that day and asked me what was wrong. Holding back my tears, I proceeded to tell her what the doctor had told me. She said, "Dad, you have never been a quitter, and did not raise your children to be quitters either, so don't let anyone steal your power. There is someone out there that can heal you."

I thought, "She is right, and I am going to find that person."

I spent the next 48 hours searching everything I could about stem cells and started to get an education on the different kinds available. And then I ran across your website. My gut feeling was, "Dr. Rader is the man I need to put my trust in."

Naturally I was anxious to get this done ASAP, since this problem had been going on for almost three years. I called your office and scheduled the next available appointment.

Within one week after I received the fetal cells, I started to notice that my energy was increasing and that the pressure in my legs and feet had let up a little. My calf muscles were still hurting, and there was no noticeable difference in the paralysis in my right leg and foot.

Two weeks after I was treated, I went to the gym for the first time in a very long time. I focused on my feet, calves, and thighs. I thought I did pretty well, but not great. However, I made my mind up that I would soon do great; it was just around the corner.

The breakthrough came at approximately one month post treatment. Where before, I had such weakness from the paralysis in my right foot, I now for the first time noticed a little muscle strength when I pushed off to go up some stairs. I had not had that feeling for three years! My feet were still burning a bit and were still numb, but there was definitely less pressure in them.

A week later I went back to gym and continued the exercises that I mentioned previously and walked a mile and a half. When I got back home I became very excited; I noticed small muscles beginning to form in my right and left calf. That was when I knew I had to shift gears and keep the power flowing.

The next week, I went to the gym, went home, and walked another one-and-a-half miles. When I got home, for the first time in three years my calf muscles were not hurting nearly as much. Oh, happy day!

So without boring you with every day's agenda, I want you to know I am continuing to walk and go to the gym, and my legs are feeling much, much better. I am so excited to be walking with not only almost no pain, but also, I am getting my muscles back!

And by the way, you are the man. I know you have to be extremely proud of what you have made available for me and others whom doctors have told, "You have no hope." Well, I now know without a doubt there is hope for the many that would put their trust in you. Therefore, I really, really believe that what you have done for me will ultimately lead me to a complete recovery. I know it's just a matter of time.

I apologize to you for such a lengthy e-mail, but I am so excited, and you will never know how blessed I feel to have had the privilege to be one of your patients. You are a powerful and compassionate doctor, unlike most I've ever met.

Always know that I am here for you in anything and everything.
Peace to you and yours.

Dear Dr. Rader,

I want to again share with you Jonathan's medical history. During the 36th week of my pregnancy, the OB noticed a problem with my baby, so he did an ultrasound and immediately referred us to a specialist. The specialist told us that Jonathan had severe holoprosencephaly, a congenital anomaly in which there is incomplete development of his brain and that it wasn't likely that he would survive his birth. And if he did live, he would be a vegetable.

Jonathan survived. An MRI confirmed the diagnosis of severe holoprosencephaly as well as hydrocephalus, a condition in which excess fluid builds up in the brain

When we went to you for the stem cells, my firm wish was for the stem cells to grow a new motor cortex in Jonathan's brain so he could gain motor skills. I just wanted him to have improved head and trunk control. I wanted him to be able to move and sit and control his hands.

Yet the stem cells had their own agenda. They wanted to become seeds of intelligence. Which is the most profound change I've noticed in Jonathan—cognitive awareness.

The baby that wasn't meant to be more than a vegetable is understanding the world around him more and more, beginning to find himself and discover his individuality, and wishes to improve himself. Since his treatment Jonathan continues to make miraculous progress. He has gained awareness of the order of things—first we do this, then we do that. He understands me when I talk to him. He understands words and expressions. He has a newfound wish to try things. He knows what he wants and how to get it. Jonathan is finding new and different ways to communicate with us. Before the cells, he had very minimal comprehension.

Today, he understands, for example, when I ask him to wait while I go to get his bottle. He can recognize and distinguish many objects, like car and ball and dog and many more. He knows when we say, "Let's go to the park," and when we're going to go out to the store. If we don't have him out of the house by 5 p.m. he lets us know he is displeased. Also he is very motivated when he sees other children. In the past he would ignore them. Now he starts kicking and moving and shrieking to get their attention.

He laughs at all sorts of things, children playing, dogs running around. He'll be watching something and then throw his head back in laughter.

It almost feels like the stem cells were the initial construction workers that were clearing the debris of a site and working on creating a space for a stronger foundation. The stem cells knew there was a natural order. They knew Jonathan needed this self awareness, this curiosity, for him to have the wish to improve his own motor skills. And with this foundation, we are now seeing great improvements in his physical abilities.

Jonathan had an MRI this morning. Here are the comparisons:

The first MRI was performed in November 6, 2006; before he received the fetal stem cells (he received them twice). The second MRI was performed today, July 10, 2009. This was about as close as I could find in terms of view so you could compare apples to apples. The hydrocephalus has resolved.

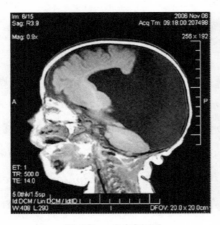

#1 Nov. 06 2006   #2 July 10, 2009

It's miraculous how much Jonathan's brain has grown from the stem cells. It's amazing!

In 1979 at the age of 27, I was first diagnosed with Type 1 Diabetes. I was admitted to the hospital because of DKA. (Diabetic ketoacidosis), a potentially life-threatening complication in patients with diabetes).

When I was discharged, the doctor told me I had to calculate the exact dose of insulin I would take before every meal, for the rest of my life.

Even being very careful, my blood sugar never would consistently get under control and I was in and out of the hospital two or three times every month with my sugar instead of being normal at 100, it was as lows as 15 and as high as 700 to 1000.

Finally in 2005, my doctors felt they were at a loss as to what more they could do, so they referred me to the Mayo Clinic. At the Mayo Clinic they told me that I needed a pancreas transplant, that my pancreas was dying and unable to produce insulin.

From the end of 2005 till April of 2009, I would fly to the Mayo Clinic and stay a month or sometimes, even longer. My blood sugar became so bad that it would either drop or go up within a blink of an eye, right in front of the nurses.

All the doctors and nurses couldn't believe how out of control it was. I began to feel that I was looked upon by the staff as a hopeless patient that was going to die.

Between visits to Mayo, I averaged 3 to 4 times a week having to go to the emergency room, because of my blood sugar being completely out of control.

It got to the point where all my friends wouldn't call, for it was the same old thing, over and over, either I was in the hospital, or in the emergency room.

By 2009 the Mayo Clinic had completely given up on me and even took me off the transplant list. But my loving husband was unwilling to give up. For the next six months he was on the computer day and night looking for something that could help me and then he finally discovered stem cells.

He called a doctor in Costa Rica about me getting my own cells, with a bone marrow stem cell transplant. We sent them my records and about two weeks later they called back with the bad news: I needed stronger stem cells than they could give me and that they were very sorry, but they were unable to help.

Well that was the final straw. My mind went crazy, I knew my life was over, and I would be without my loving family before too long. I just gave up, hung my head, and wanted to be left alone. While I was still upset, the phone rang. It was one of Dr. Rader's staff returning my husband's email inquiry.

Suddenly my mood completely changed and I felt that this telephone call could be Gods way of giving me back the gift of life. We scheduled the next available treatment.

The first time I met Dr. Rader and his staff, I was amazed, for it had felt as though I had known them, for all of my life, just fantastic people.

When I returned to the airport, after my treatment and was waiting for my plane home, I started to feel something, a rush of energy starting to flow in my body. I wasn't just wishing. It really was happening. It actually felt weird, feeling so good, after I had been so down and dragging, for such a long period of time.

I was starting to GET LIFE BACK INTO ME, and so soooooon.

A day after I got home, I started to gain control of my blood sugar.

Today my blood sugar is stable, using only one dose of insulin a day. I no longer have those life threatening ups and downs, where I would end up in the hospital emergency room. I haven't had to go to the emergency room, not even once!

I feel really, really good and I have gotten my energy and strength back.

All thanks to our DEAR FATHER and thank you Dr. Rader and staff.

We love you.

Dear Dr. Rader,

This letter is to give you an update on my 17-year-old daughter Annette, who suffers from Charcot-Marie-Tooth disease.

First I would like to tell you about her prior to her treatment three years ago. The disease affected her from her knees down to her toes, and from her elbow to her hands, and she had severe muscle atrophy due to the nerve damage.

Prior to treatment, Annette would always push herself to do the things other kids her age were doing. She would push so hard that by 8 o'clock every evening she would need to be in bed to rest for the next day. If she went swimming or did any physical activity, it would take several days for her body to not feel fatigued.

I was told that when she walked, it was as if each of her legs weighed an extra 15 lbs, and when she would try to walk up stairs, the weight of each of her legs increased to an extra 30 lbs.!

After her initial treatment, the first three weeks or so, from time to time she would show a burst of energy, and then she would need to lie down and rest. After the six-week period the energy never stopped. She was full of life like we have never seen before.

You told us to keep her active, so we enrolled her with a personal trainer twice a week, 30 minutes each session. What we started to see was unbelievable. We noticed that she would walk up the stairs to the house more often then she would crawl, like she had to for so many years. She now walks down them as well, instead of sliding down. We have seen her catch herself when she falls instead of falling on her face, which in the past has often happened.

At school she was allotted extra time get to her classes, but now she doesn't need it anymore, because she is able to walk fast enough to get to class like everyone else.

Currently, not only does she work with a personal trainer two times a week, she takes water aerobics, lifts weights, and attends spinning classes with me. On the cycle, she will peddle for 45 minutes and still have enough energy to leave the gym and go do other things like walking at the mall. She has slimmed down and, with a great deal of confidence, excitedly carries forward every day when she wakes up.

Keep in mind that prior to the stem cells there was no way Annette could have done any type of exercising whatsoever and then been able to get up and go to school the next day. It would have taken her days to recuperate. The fetal stem cell treatment has not only made a dramatic life change for her, but also has allowed me to finally have peace of mind about her future.

I am so proud of her. She is finishing the eighth grade with A–B grades, and she is arranging her high school schedule to be able, at the same time, to take college classes.

What an inspiration for other people to see and what a story to tell! Because of her experience, Annette has decided to become a nurse.

And most of all, I thank you, Dr. Rader. I am looking forward to what she will be doing next. Maybe someday you two will be working together!

Dear Dr. Rader,

I have had lupus since 1983. The symptoms I have are inflammation of the lining of lungs and heart along with pleurisy. The inflammation and pleurisy cause severe chest pain and shortness of breath.

In 1994, my attacks became more frequent. My doctor did a treatment called apheresis (blood separation) and began chemotherapy using Cytoxan. The chemotherapy was done on an as-needed basis. In the beginning the Cytoxan treatments were pretty frequent, but eventually I was able to go three to six months between Cytoxan treatments.

In December of 2007, I began to have attacks with intense chest pains. As usual, my doctor ordered the Cytoxan treatment. This was the beginning of my nightmare. For some reason, my body decided to reject the treatment. From that point on, the Cytoxan treatments did nothing to stop the pain. From December to May, they tried everything they thought could possibly help, including more apheresis treatments and Solu-Medrol drips. Nothing worked.

Meanwhile, my doctor was performing all types of tests to see if they could determine the cause of the attacks. My attacks in the past could usually be pinpointed to something else going on, such as flu, colds, infections, etc. Nothing showed up on any of the tests. He told me there was nothing more he could do and that most probably I would continue to suffer from intensely painful uncontrollable lupus attacks.

In May 2008, I thought it could not get any worse, but then it did. I no longer had any strength due to the high dosages of steroids and the painful attacks. I was taking from 40 mg to 60 mg of prednisone a day just to try to lessen the pain. My legs became so weak that I could not step up onto a curb without falling. The chest pains were so severe that just trying to breathe was becoming more and more difficult. The doctors were unable to find anything to lessen my attacks.

I now knew that I was dying.

I had been talking to Medra for several months and was preparing to make their June treatment date, but then, as I rapidly got weaker and weaker, I knew I would not be able to live much longer, so I made arrangements for the next available treatment.

I received my fetal stem cells Saturday, May 3, 2008. I woke up the next morning completely pain free, and I have remained so since. Three weeks after my stem cell treatment, I went for a follow-up appointment with my rheumatologist. He was just amazed by my lack of symptoms. He decided to run a complete blood work on me. When he got the results back, he called me and said he was "stunned." Everything was basically normal. He told me I was in remission.

All my relatives and friends are happily astounded. I have no chest pain at all, and I can feel myself getting stronger and stronger day by day. I can even easily walk up steps.

I thank God every day for the stem cell procedure and that I am still alive.

Medra received this letter from the parents of a young woman who was paralyzed in a traffic accident:

On October 31, 2004, my daughter, who was nine months pregnant, was in an SUV rollover. She suffered a C4-C5 spinal cord injury and was left paralyzed from the neck down. The baby survived with extensive brain damage. The doctors all suggested I put my daughter in an institution so that she could get 24/7 care, since she was not going to get better. They did not even bother to give her any therapy, for it was a waste of time, according to them.

Four years after the accident, my daughter was only able to move her left arm; she could not feel anything else in her body. It was at that time I came across Dr. Rader's web site.

We had the stem cell therapy in 2008, and she started to feel different parts of her body. After a couple of months she was able to feel her legs, her right arm started moving more, her overall heath improved, and her memory got clearer.

We were very pleased and decided to return for a second treatment in June 2009, and this time we took her daughter to get the stem cells, too. My granddaughter has extensive brain damage, and at the age of four she can't sit, crawl, talk, or even hold her head up. She is legally blind and being fed by a feeding tube.

We recently got back from the procedure, and to our amazement she is showing good progress also. In her physical therapy they have noticed a big improvement in her movement and her attention span. She is also starting to hold her head up on her own. The therapist has clocked her holding her head on her own for nine minutes; that in itself is amazing.

We could not be happier and look forward to seeing more improvements in both of them. We thank Dr. Rader and his staff for providing hope to us parents where the medical community didn't see any.

Dear Dr. Rader,

I appreciate all the help you have given Jerry and myself. The treatments are definitely working for Jerry's pulmonary fibrosis (scarring of the lung). Jerry can breathe 75 percent better. His lips are no longer blue, and his skin has much more color. He hasn't had to get a breathing treatment or inhalers since he got the stem cells. The day after treatment we had to walk almost a mile in the airport to get to our ride in Orlando. He was able to do that without stopping. Yay!!!! Jerry is actually working in the yard, something he has not been able to do for years. The chronic obstructive pulmonary disease is not winning this fight.

On the other hand, as you know, I have a diagnosis of heart disease, asthma, and sleep apnea. I too have been breathing much better, and I have a lot more energy. I'm able to chase my German shepherd puppies around the yard. Also, my outlook on life has improved. My skin is healing; normally I end up with scars because of taking Plavix.

I realize we are blessed to be able to be treated. Most people are not that fortunate.

I truly wish your treatment doesn't go unnoticed. I know it has saved many, including children, from deadly diseases.

The following is from the mother of a young patient diagnosed with Cockayne Syndrome (CS) II, a rare genetic disorder characterized by growth failure and other abnormalities apparent at birth.

My daughter Susan was 5 years old when she first received the definite diagnoses of Cockayne Syndrome (CS) Type II in August of 2007. CS is a very rare, neurodegenerative disease characterized by cataracts at birth, developmental delays, tremors, failure to thrive and loss of major milestones. The most devastating thing about CS is that Susan's life expectancy was only between 4 and 7 years old.

Susan had begun to have tremors by age 2 1/2 and by the age of 3 1/2 she was completely unable to walk any longer. With the help of her walker she was able to get around a bit. She has been on numerous medications for the tremors and her sleeping problems and her reflux. We finally found a Parkinson's medication that improved her tremors a bit, but Susan is too small to be given a higher dose and she gets an adverse reaction to an increase in dosage. As for sleeping, Susan had been on everything from Benadryl to heavy narcotics, all to no avail. So far there is no treatment or cure for CS. All I could do was to keep trying new medications to help Susan function better.

In April of 2008 our world changed forever. We were introduced to someone who told us about stem cell therapy and how well it had worked for his son. Although quite skeptical, I was feeling a bit of hope that this treatment could also benefit my daughter. I spoke to Dr. Rader

125

and soon after that in May of 2008, Susan had her first stem cell treatment. At that time she was almost 6 years old and very shaky, not even able to pull herself up to a standing position. By the time we went for her second treatment in October 2008, there was a definite decrease in Susan's tremors and her attention span in school had gotten much better.

After her second stem cell treatment Susan's tremors were even more significantly reduced and she was becoming more and more attentive in school. She was also able to walk longer distances with her walker and had more energy. Although Susan can't say too many words, she now was using many more sounds and approximations to make her needs known.

The third treatment was in April of 2009 and this was the miracle treatment for Susan! In about June 2009 Susan began sleeping through the night 10 hours at a time without any medication! Even with all of the sleeping medication we had tried, Susan hadn't slept through a night in 4 years!!! At this time she also began going on the potty and now will let me know whenever she needs to go! She was also beginning to try to stand independently for 10-20 seconds at a time and pulling up on the refrigerator to open it and unlocking and opening the front door! She now wants to do everything herself! Susan turned 7 in August 2009. The few CS Type II children who actually live until 7 are usually very, very sick by then and are certainly not gaining any new milestones. To our amazement, two weeks after her 7th birthday, Susan took her first independent steps in almost 4 years!! She walked very slow and steady taking steps for the camera and has continued to try to take steps everyday!

This is nothing short of a miracle.

I will be forever grateful to Dr. Rader for giving Susan an improved quality of life and for giving me and their mother hope. Hope for another step, another word, another birthday, hope for a future with my child.

Dr. Rader:

I want to share with you what I am going to put on Beth's web site.

Beth's Progress Report

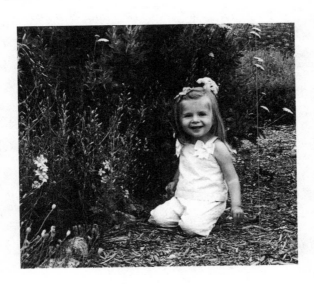

Spinal Muscular Atrophy

Spinal muscular atrophy (SMA) is a genetic disease resulting in a progressive loss of motor neurons of the brainstem and spinal cord. Children with SMA do not improve—they only regress.

The onset is sudden and dramatic. Once symptoms occur, the motor neuron cells quickly deteriorate. The earlier the symptoms appear, the shorter the lifespan. There is no cure yet known. Spinal muscular atrophy can be fatal.

Motor Skills Prior to Becoming Sick

Beth reached all of her normal milestones up until nine months of age. She rolled, got herself into a sitting position, crawled, stood, and took steps around a table and also with her toy walker. And she could walk four passes on the monkey bars.

At 16 months of age suddenly everything changed.

- *Beth could not crawl. She was unable to even roll over. If we placed her on all fours, she did not have the muscle strength to hold her position without collapsing.*

- *She could not pick up her foot to take a step. The doctors told us our beautiful daughter was not expected to ever take a step again in her life.*

- *She lost the ability to even reach her hand up to her mouth.*

- *She became so floppy that picking her up under her arms be-came very difficult.*

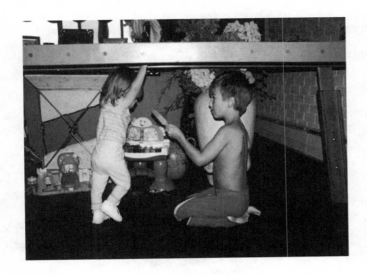

Stem Cell Treatment #1: 10/26/07

- *Instead of getting worse, as was expected in a SMA child, Beth began to regain muscle strength and get better.*
- *Now, for the first time since she became ill, she was able to pick up her legs and walk four feet holding onto a table.*
- *She was much less floppy under the arms and easier to pick up.*

Stem Cell Treatment #2: 2/22/08

- *Beth can walk a number of steps with her toy walker now.*
- *She can reach over her head.*
- *She can stay on all fours by herself.*
- *She walks six rungs on the monkey bars.*
- *She is even able to stand independently.*

Stem Cell Treatment #3: 5/31/08

- *Beth walked a full pass on the monkey bars (10 feet).*

- *She now has the strength to push a dresser drawer closed.*
- *She can now walk over 30 feet with her toy walker.*

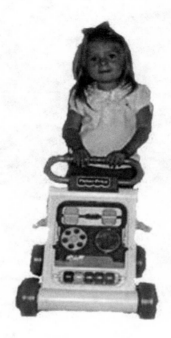

Stem Cell Treatment #4, 9/27/08

- *Beth took two steps without hanging on to anything.*
- *She is able to walk two passes on the monkey bars.*
- *She can walk 100 feet while just hanging on to someone's fingers.*

We were told that our child would never be able to walk again, that she would continually get worse and that there was nothing known that could stop her deadly decline.

We can never thank you enough, Dr. Rader, for proving them wrong!

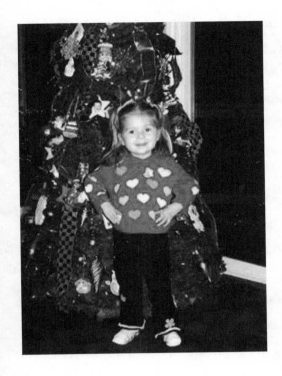

*Look at me. I'm standing **<u>all by myself</u>**.*

Thanks to you, Dr. Rader!!

Dr. Rader,

I wanted to write you and thank you for saving my life. The results of that one treatment of fetal stem cells that I received over four years ago have proved to be nothing short of a miracle. At that time, my kidneys were in such bad shape that the doctors were preparing to start me on hemodialysis, with an eye toward an eventual kidney transplant.

I am no longer having any signs or symptoms of my polycystic kidney disease, which, as you know, is always supposed to be progressive, to the point of destroying all kidney function.

At the present time and since shortly after I was treated four years ago, all my laboratory results, including my creatinine levels, have continued to be within the normal range.

By William C. Rader, MD

The stem cells have also relieved many joint pains that I was experiencing prior to receiving the treatment, and my body also seems to have the ability to heal itself better after injury.

I am so grateful. Thank you for the difference you have made in my life.

Dr. Rader,

For some reason that I cannot explain, I have had a series of medical misfortunes throughout my life. First and foremost was my rheumatoid arthritis. Prior to the stem cell treatment, my day was over the minute I could drag myself home from my desk job, which took all my energy. Extreme fatigue is one of the main symptoms of rheumatoid arthritis. I could only plop down in a chair, and would eat only if my husband prepared and served dinner. It was all I could do. I'd have to call it a day and go straight to bed to sleep immediately afterwards. If dinner wasn't presented to me, I just wouldn't eat. And sometimes I was too tired to eat anyway.

In the weeks and months following the treatment, I have become increasingly energized. Now I not only enjoy preparing dinner, but I shop for ingredients on the way home, do the dishes afterwards, plus play with our cats, watch a movie, do chores, or anything else that comes to mind. I do whatever I want, whenever I want.

My husband and I go out evenings and on the weekends, even outside, which used to drain me so quickly. Now I can even garden.

We have once again become active in community activities, social and entertainment opportunities, etc. I am much stronger, have more stamina, and oodles of energy. I actually feel peppy! I seem to be growing younger instead of older as time passes. It's like I got my life back!

Something I find amazing is how I am now able to stay warm instead of feeling like I'm freezing all the time, indoors and out. I was the icicle-fingers lady with the popsicle toes and nose. I used an electric blanket on my bed at night, every night, year-round. It was set on medium in the summer and high all winter, spring, and fall. Even when sitting around at home, I had a heated throw across my lap. I have always used these electric blankets for as far back as I can remember; I have not used any since my treatment, and I'm just fine. I stay plenty warm and comfortable by myself. I now have a metabolism that is running warmer and keeping me comfortable and healthier in general.

Another major change is that my fetal stem cell infusion has allowed me to finally stop regular chiropractic treatment, after decades of weekly treatments. I'd injured my lower back decades ago and also had suffered severe whiplash in the mid 1980s. For years I had chiropractic adjustments four times per week, plus diathermy, ice packs, and other modalities of treatment that chiropractics and physical therapy have to offer. All was in an effort to reduce the severe clamping headaches caused by the whiplash and to reduce the constant, chronic pain from my low-back injury. Over the years, I'd slowly reduced my visits to the chiropractor to once a week or so, but at times I had to be back in there daily, seeking any relief possible. And most often, there was either minimal or no relief at all.

Now, since the stem cells, I have not been back to the chiropractor, not even once. Nor am I in pain. Nor am I so fragile that even a pat on the back could knock me out of alignment and send me scurrying for an adjustment.

What a great way to get my life back!

Also, in the early 1990s my left ear was injured by a very loud noise in a confined space. Ever since then there was a rattling sound inside my ear. I could not lay my left ear against a pillow or the rattling noise would become even more pronounced. There was not one day I did not experience this nagging nuisance, until now. It hasn't rattled or spasmed or whatever you what to call it since.

After five years of continuous use of Flonase for nasal congestion, I now have completely stopped using this prescription. I'm no longer noticing a stuffy nose. It's been months now. I think I'm free of my allergies at last!

A month after my return from getting my treatment, I caught a cold from my coworkers. This was the first cold I had in years that did not also include a miserable cold sore or fever blister along with it. I am convinced that stem cells really help defeat herpes, because of this and because I have only now have stopped suffering from the aftermath of a severe outbreak of shingles on my leg.

Since that episode of shingles four years ago, my leg had not been free from pain along the three nerve tracks that the shingles had appeared on. I thought it would bother me for the rest of my life, as many people had told me that theirs did after they had shingles. But it doesn't bother me anymore since my treatment. I'm free from yet more chronic pain.

With all of my medical symptoms, I would wonder sometimes if I was just a chronic complainer or even, as some described me, a hypochondriac. But now that they're all gone, I know that they were real.

Every day I continue to be amazed about how good I feel. I'm normal!!

1/9/2009 Linda's Progress

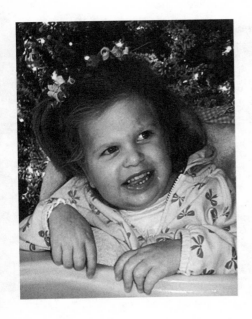

1. *Hurray! Linda, for the first time since her brain injury, has movement in her right side; she is even able to move her right arm and pull up her right leg.*
2. *Linda's right hand was always in a tight fist. Now it has become loose. And when she stretches, her fingers are completely straight.*
3. *Her appetite has continued to increase, allowing her to gain weight.*

4. *Before the stem cells, Linda usually was sleeping by 3 to 4 in the afternoon and would stay asleep until the next morning. Now she has a lot of energy. She even stayed up till 12 midnight for New Year's!*

5. *Ever since her brain injury, her eyes would rapidly flutter back and forth all the time without ever stopping. Her nystagmus has now completely disappeared!*

6. *Her pupils are much more reactive to light and dark. Prior to the treatment, there was very little response.*

7. *We have seen an overall reduction in her seizures. She used to have 2 to 4 major seizures a day, lasting approximately 3 to 5 minutes (myoclonic type), and now she, at worst, may have one very quick minor seizure-like event a night.*

8. *Linda is trying to talk so-o-o-o hard. She is pushing air and moving her mouth to say a word. We know she is close to talking and we are so excited!*

9. *Linda has been able to go to the bathroom without the use of a laxative. Prior to the treatment, Linda always had to receive multiple laxatives.*

10. *Around 8:30 p.m. on January 7th, Linda put her left thumb in her mouth and was just moving it around slightly. Then she started to suck her thumb. This went on for about 10 seconds. This may not sound like a major achievement, but for my little angel, after all the doctors had given me no hope for any recovery, for us it was a milestone. I was overcome with emotion, and just couldn't stop crying. This is truly another sign that the stem cells are working.*

Last night on my way home from work, I prayed to God about my Linda and once again asked for His help and guidance in healing her (as I do several times throughout my day, every day). But this time it was different. I spoke with God out loud to show myself, here, in my reality, that He has heard my prayers. He not only does, but He is answering them.

Dear Dr. Rader,

I can't tell you how thrilled both my husband and I are with the results of the fetal stem cell treatments my husband has received. Approximately six and a half years ago John received the diagnosis of primary lateral sclerosis PLS, a rare neuromuscular disease characterized by progressive muscle weakness in the voluntary muscles. His doctor told us that there was nothing that mainstream medicine could do for him. Thus began our research into alternative treatments.

After researching and trying several different avenues, we had a rather serendipitous meeting with a couple whose child had received fetal stem cell treatments and his condition was improving immensely. Without the fetal stem cell treatments, he most likely would have died from his condition.

We then began looking into stem cell treatments for John. After having done quite a bit of research on our own, John had a consultation with Dr. Rader. The research itself was compelling, but the sincerity of the doctor and the results of so many of his patients spurred us into action.

John has now received two fetal stem cell treatments over a one-year period. Not only has the PLS ceased to progress, but the improvement in his gait, fine motor movements, and speech has been nothing less than miraculous.

Needless to say, Dr. Rader and the fetal stem cell treatments have offered us hope in an arena where there was little and more quality of life than John had ever hoped to regain.

Dear Dr. Rader,

As I shared with you, as a professional opera singer it was devastating for me to realize I was losing my voice. I want you to know that this week my voice teacher told me I had progressed five years in three months.

I received your therapy three months ago. When I sing for my boss now, he hugs me and tells me, "That was beautiful."

I have not been sick one time since then. My strength is returning. I am singing better than ever in my entire life. I wanted to thank you again and say God bless you. You are doing wondrous things.

The next time I have a recital I will send you tickets, should you wish to attend.

Dr. Rader

I'm writing to tell you about what a terrific experience I've had as a result of being able to receive the fetal stem cell therapy.

In November of 2002, I contacted you and asked about the stem cell therapy you were doing. My concerns were longevity, anti-aging, improving my immune system, and improving the quality of my skin. You agreed that the stem cells could be a benefit to me and I came for a treatment that month.

After waiting the three to six month period for the stem cells to become most effective, I didn't notice any difference in the way I looked or the way I felt. When I voiced my concerns to you, you told me that the cells must be working on something that I wasn't aware of, but just to be sure you suggested I come back for another dose.

I returned in May of 2003. In June of 2004 I was diagnosed with chronic lymphocytic leukemia. My internist thought that without my having the stem cells, there was a chance that the leukemia could have been acute instead of chronic. If it had turned to acute, it may have been fatal.

I decided to have the stem cells again after my diagnosis. My latest blood test showed that instead of one third of my cells being atypical (as they were when I was first diagnosed), I had absolutely no atypical cells. I no longer have leukemia. I have been given a totally clean bill of health.

The lab that reported the test results to my internist had remarked that they had never seen this happen before.

You have been a tremendous support to me during this entire time. I am so very, very grateful for all your help and caring.

P.S. Also the quality of my skin now is terrific.

Dear Dr. Rader,

I wanted to take this opportunity to say how thankful I am that you are in our lives. You mean so much to me and Mark, and I felt this Christmas was the perfect chance to tell you.

By William C. Rader, MD

Eleven years ago, when Mark was only four months old (12/11/97), he developed an aneurysm which ruptured. He died three times and was resuscitated three times. His medical records say that his brain was anoxic-hypoxic for 30 to 45 minutes, and I was given no hope. After a few days, his condition began to stabilize, and he was weaned from life support. Ten days after he first bled into his brain, his aneurysm ruptured for a second time. This time it was determined to be about three times the amount of blood as the first bleed, and they gave him 24 hours to live.

They had us plan his funeral, and they even described to us what his last breath would look like. It was the most painful moment of my life. Then, unexpectedly, he began to stabilize again and remained in what the doctors called a semi-vegetative state. Although we were given no hope for any type of recovery for Mark, I refused to give up on my son and began my search for anything that could possibly help.

After two years of constant searching, using everything I could find, from the Internet to medical journals, I heard about stem cells. I began researching and digging to determine if stem cells could possibly help Mark. I eventually found Medra.

In the summer of 2000, we first met you, and it has been the best thing I could have possibly done for Mark. I believe the Lord used you to save Mark's life. It is during this time of year, as you know, that I write you to once again thank you for what you continue to do for my son, and I want you to know how grateful I really am. We always cry and marvel at how far my sweet boy has come. He continues to improve, in spite of all the hopeless and negative medical predictions I was given from that scary rough start.

We continue to see his personality develop, and every day he understands more and more of what we say to him. His vision also continues to improve. He has gone from 20/2700 to recently being tested at 20/470.

His quality of life has changed drastically. You can see the little person inside emerging. I have you to thank for that. This is by far, the greatest gift of all—seeing my lovely son continue to get better.

After each treatment we seem to always see bigger changes. His brain is being rebuilt from the ground floor up. Also, his seizures have significantly reduced in number and intensity. When we first came to see you he suffered with over 500 major seizures a day, and now he is down to only about 10 very minor seizure-like episodes.

One very special trait you have is that you believe. You were the only one of all the professionals who took a chance to believe in Mark, and you treated him like a person and not a "fixture." The treatment you give is giving my son life, hope for a future, and I know he now believes in himself.

He works so hard in therapy, and he just amazes everyone. I think that it is because he is encouraged, because he knows he is getting better all the time.

You dared to believe that you could fight the system and offer fetal stem cell treatments that could so dramatically change lives. And you continue to believe in and support the hopeful parents, who were given no hope at all for their child.

We truly love you and pray for your health and safety.

By William C. Rader, MD

Scleroderma, which afflicted the subject of the following letter, is a chronic disease characterized by a hardening or sclerosis in the skin or other organs. There is no cure for scleroderma. Any treatment is aimed only at ameliorating symptoms. Scleroderma can be fatal, as a result of heart, kidney, lung or intestinal damage.

Dr. Rader,

Alan had his stem cell transplant on the 26th for his systemic scleroderma. All of us were hopeful, but at the same time very nervous! Anyway, everything went very well— the staff was great! Alan noticed changes almost immediately. The next morning he was able to move the fingers on his left hand, and by that evening he could even hold a glass with it—absolutely remarkable!

Over the next few days, there were more advancements as well. He now has no knee pain. (Because of his scleroderma, one of his knees used to continually pop in and out of place). He has not choked for two days now. He has no joint pain in general. Amazingly, he has been losing those awful calcium deposits from his hands. We are hopeful the ones on his armpits and butt will be next.

In a nutshell, everything is going great. We are very grateful for finding out about Medra and then taking the big leap to get Alan treated.

Dear Dr. Rader

I wanted to take a moment to let you know how happy my husband and I are with the results of our son's stem cell treatment. Our two year old son Bobby was diagnosed with Menkes Disease, a genetic neurodegenerative brain disorder which has resulted in our precious little child being severely developmentally delayed and having very weak muscle tone.

Children with Menkes Disease are not supposed to live past the age of three. Since receiving his treatment, instead of him getting worse, as all of his doctors had predicted, we are seeing marked improvements. Every day he continues to show advancements both physically and cognitively. Bobby has gained weight, grown in length and even his head circumference has grown. He feeds by mouth and now chews. He no longer is only on formula but can eat table foods. He is now able to hold his head up and move it from side to side. He has flexion throughout his spine and can roll over and kick his toys. He traces you with his eyes and follows and mimics sounds.

Recently, one of the biggest changes has been the development of strong muscles throughout his entire body. We continue to be full of hope for Bobby. With the help of the fetal stem cells there is no limitation to what we feel our son can accomplish.

Doctor Rader,

Just a few hours after my son Robert was treated for his cerebral palsy, I was virtually levitating with excitement because of the miracles I was seeing. For the first time in his life, my sweet little boy was able to take reciprocating steps. Usually he drags both feet together when he's in his walker. But minutes after the fetal stem cell shot, he was able to take regular steps in his walker with his feet flat on the floor. In the past he always stood on tippy toes and couldn't place his feet flat on the floor. He even stopped having spasms. It brought tears to my eyes when he said to me, "Mommy, I'm not spasming any more." Then he began to show off a bunch of his new skills. He could move his wrists and hands in circles. He took a paper and pen and started to draw circles for the first time. He was able to move his arms and hands effortlessly. His body was relaxed and his adductors were loose.

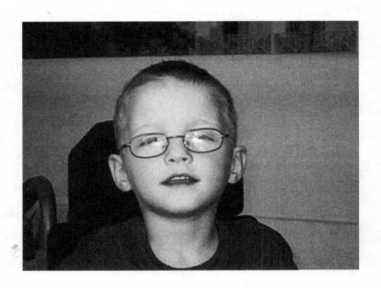

All through that first day and night he proudly showed us all the new things that he had been unable to do just the day before.

That first night right before he went to bed he said, "Dr. Rader fixed me!"

Aging and Longevity

Let's face it—we're all getting older. And while it may seem far less dire than the other afflictions discussed in this book, aging is the one "disease" we all share—at least all of us fortunate enough to live to middle age and beyond.

Moreover, for many of us, aging happens faster than necessary because in today's world we're beset by factors such as high stress, poor diet, and environmental toxins, all of which contribute to chronic diseases not part of the natural aging process.

Americans spend billions on cosmetic, health, and diet products, and large sums are spent on scientific research, all in the quest to halt the aging process and discover the fountain of youth. Yet nothing I know of does more to stave off aging and preserve youthful vitality than fetal stem cell therapy.

The body's cells are programmed to replicate themselves approximately 60 to 80 times, and each time cellular reproduction occurs, the cells' telomeres become shorter—telomeres being the protective arms that defend chromosomes and the genetic structure within them.

As I previously noted, fetal stem cells contain fully intact, original-length telomeres, as well as an abundance of telomerase, the enzyme responsible for producing telomeres. This is a principal factor in the ability of fetal stem cells to help the body ward off toxins and pathogens and to rejuvenate the body's organ systems.

After fetal stem cell therapy, patients consistently report clearer thought, improved memory, higher energy and optimism about life, and cosmetic benefits that include firmer skin tone, diminution of wrinkles, decreased body fat, increased lean muscle, and occasionally even hair growth. It is common for my female patients to be asked if they've had a facelift.

First and foremost, our bodies are designed for procreation—to keep passing on our genetic material. The body is genetically programmed to grow and become more robust until it reaches prime reproductive age. As that period passes, the body slowly begins to degenerate. However, when fetal stem cells are introduced into an adult body, they do what they are programmed to do: act as if the adult were a large, damaged fetus that needs to be repaired and maintained to maximize its ability to procreate.

Fetal stem cells act generically in repairing and maintaining the body. That is, after entering the body, they seek out cells, tissues, and organs that have any level of damage.

Initially, as I explained previously, the fetal stem cells release cytokines, which stimulate the body's own repair mechanisms. Then, over time, the fetal stem cells repair and/or create any of the body's 220 cell types.

In my experience, this repair-and-replacement process includes a kind of triage effect, in which the tissues most in need of repair get it first. It also plays a major role in controlling both localized and systemic inflammation, which are now seen as major factors in many age-related degenerative diseases, including heart disease and certain types of cancer.

The bottom line is this: Fetal stem cell therapy triggers a generalized "youthening" effect, repairing and rejuvenating cells, tissues, and organs.

A Stronger Immune System

Once you know how fetal stem cells work in the body, understanding their anti-aging benefits is easy. For example, impaired immunity is a primary cause of aging—of both physical and mental decline. The immune system protects us from a host of pathogens, including cancer. The stronger our immune system remains, the more resistant we are to illness. Also, a stronger immune system promotes increased physical energy and mental clarity.

cause of aging

In general, the younger we are, the stronger our immune system is. That is one of the main reasons why children are far less likely to be stricken by serious illnesses than adults.

The likelihood of developing cancer is actually generally proportionate to the aging process. For example, breast and prostate cancer are far more common in people over 50 than they are in those in their 20s and 30s, and such cancers are virtually nonexistent among children and teens.

Every one of us develops 250 million new cancer and precancerous cells every day of our lives. When we are optimally healthy, these potentially dangerous cells do not pose a threat because they are targeted and destroyed by our immune system.

Develope cancer cells daily

But as we age, our immune system weakens, making it easier for these cells to survive and multiply. Weakened immunity also makes us more likely to contract infectious diseases and then allows these diseases to become more severe.

However, patients who receive fetal stem cells, as I noted earlier, develop a new immune system—a system that works in concert with the one they have but is at least ten times stronger than a normal healthy adult's, thereby significantly reducing the likelihood of becoming ill.

Fetal Stem Cell Therapy vs. Hormone Therapy

As the populations of developed nations have aged, a major branch of medicine, anti-aging, has emerged to help us remain healthier and more youthful. A primary goal of anti-aging medicine is to improve immune function. The strategies for reaching that objective include dietary supplements (nutritional, herbal, and others), as well as the use of natural and bio-identical hormones to restore peak hormone levels.

Fetal stem cells can accomplish the same goal, far more effectively and efficiently, endogenously (within the body) by employing nature rather than man's invention. In lieu of relying upon oral, topical, or injectable hormonal compounds to reach a balance, fetal stem cell therapy can help restore optimal hormone levels.

A number of my patients who had been using bio-identical hormone therapy chose to stop taking them after receiving the fetal stem cells because the hormone therapy was no longer needed. A patient came to me after consulting with a well-known anti-aging specialist about her recent onset of menopausal symptoms—hot flashes, mood swings, weight gain, and so on. After spending thousands of dollars on tests, she was told she'd need an extensive array of hormones and other supplements to achieve relief. Instead, she decided to receive fetal stem cells.

One month after treatment, she began to have a normal menstrual cycle and became symptom-free. (Note, however, that this is a level of response achieved only when a patient has very recently become menopausal). Subsequently, this woman requested another battery of tests from her anti-aging specialist and was told her hormone levels were now within the normal premenopausal range.

Most anti-aging specialists are excellent physicians with specialized training; they have advanced understanding not only of the need for hormone replacement, but of how to achieve a proper hormone balance through external means, including specialized diets. I strongly favor the use of nutrients and other supplements, and I am not opposed to bio-identical hormone therapy use in the proper hands.

Unfortunately, most patients have not paid nearly enough attention to proper nutrition, sensible supplementation, exercise, stress reduction, and getting adequate sleep. Because I value and preach the value of these factors, I am a bit reluctant to say this, for obvious reasons, but: even those patients who choose to ignore my advice on diet, exercise, and lifestyle still demonstrate significant improvement in their health, energy, and cognition following fetal stem cell therapy.

Unlike the scientists and researchers constantly trying to figure out better ways to use external agents, such as drugs, supplements, or hormones to manipulate the body into a healthier state, I do nothing other than administer the fetal stem cells and let nature take its course.

Strength and Conditioning

Another huge benefit of fetal stem cells is their ability to actually turn fat into lean muscle (in patients who are not significantly over-weight).

I've had a number of longevity patients with well-developed, muscular bodies who worked out as much as six days a week to maintain their physical appearance. After receiving fetal stem cells, some stopped exercising altogether—against my advice—and still generally maintained the gains they previously achieved.

Most of our patients do continue their exercise routines and report that they're now able to achieve the same results with a lighter, shorter workout than before. Others continue to work out at their previous level and report greater results.

Cognitive Function

Some of my longevity patients are highly successful, creative, driven entertainment professionals who, as they've aged, feel they have hit a "creative wall."

Invariably, after receiving treatment, they report that their creativity and problem-solving abilities are enhanced; they feel calmer, less prone to distraction, and haven't been as productive in years.

They also describe a general feeling of well being. They just "feel good" more often than they did before—not in the sense of a euphoric "high," but in that peaceful, uncomplicated state they recall from their childhood. They are more able and more eager to be problem solvers, not worriers, and find it easier to respond to challenges.

I cannot fully explain this phenomenon, but it could be that fetal stem cells help restore healthy brain function, limiting tendencies toward depression, attention deficit, compulsive thoughts, anxiety, and so on.

The brain has a finite number of brain cells. As an analogy, let's compare those cells to a given number of soldiers in an army. Sending troops on missions unrelated to the overall campaign reduces the chances of ultimate success.

As adults, we devote a great deal of time and effort on thoughts, feelings and the like that are counterproductive to our primary agenda, such as "I'm afraid people will notice I'm not as sharp as I used to be." The brain has to devote a number of its cells (troops) to those distracting thoughts, thereby lessening the total number of brain cells (attention) that can be devoted to the task at hand.

✳ In essence, the fetal stem cells seem to quiet that part of one's inner voice that is inappropriately negative.

My Mother: A Case History

My mother Edith passed away at the age of 99. She was always very sharp mentally. Throughout her life, her intelligence and cognitive skills were very much in evidence.

When she entered her 80s, her mental acuity began to lessen slightly and her voice weakened. Then suddenly, over a two-week period, she became extremely forgetful and began to imagine things that hadn't occurred, such as visits from friends and relatives she hadn't seen for ages. Although I never told her she was imagining things, she still had the presence of mind to realize on her own that her cognitive abilities had become impaired. She had always declined my offers of fetal stem cell therapy, but now she finally agreed.

About two weeks after she received the cells, while I was traveling outside the country, I received a message on my hotel answering machine. It happened to be my birthday, and when I played the message back I heard a female voice singing "Happy Birthday." At first I thought it was my daughter because the voice was so strong and energetic. After playing it back again, I realized it was my mother.

After receiving the fetal stem cells, her cognitive abilities returned completely, and they remained unimpaired until her death more than a decade later.

My Own Experience with Fetal Stem Cell Therapy

Although there wasn't any medical reason for doing so, I decided to experience the fetal stem cell treatment for myself. As I was receiving the treatment I happened to glance at my tweed jacket hanging on a coat rack in the corner of the room. I became acutely aware of its thread pattern, which jumped out at me in sharp definition, almost what you experience watching a 3-D movie. In fact, everything came into sharp focus as I experienced a heightened level of visual acuity.

To validate my perceived experience of improved vision, I went to my optometrist for an eye exam. I didn't tell him I'd received fetal stem cells. On my last visit, years before, my eyesight had been 20/50. After measuring my vision, my optometrist expressed amazement. Instead of declining with age, as is normal, my eyesight had improved. It was now 20/15—better than normal.

A corollary to this: One of my patients was a physician who always wore glasses. After receiving fetal stem cells, he became concerned because his vision started to blur. He then was shocked to discover that, when he took off his glasses, he was able to see clearly without them. He hasn't put them on since, and it's been over three years.

Getting back to my own history. Throughout my life I've been fortunate enough to have good reflexes. If something would fall I would see it in my hand without realizing that I had reached out to catch it. Apparently I had lost that ability only becoming aware of it after the fetal stem cells when I once again had the same experience.

Getting thru all those years of "higher" education, I feel I have a very good memory, yet after receiving the fetal stem cells I am able to recall even the most obscure of things without any effort. I noticed this a few weeks after my first treatment. I was trying to recall someone's name but couldn't. I stopped trying and became involved in something else. Then, out of nowhere, a name popped into my head in a way I had never experienced before.

My first thought was, "Why am I thinking of that name?"

My second was, "Oh, now I remember. I was trying to think of someone's name."

My third was that I was positive the name that came into my mind was the wrong name. After checking further, I eventually found that the name was indeed correct.

That indicates how far away from my conscious mind the recalled memory was. It was a way of remembering that I had never experienced before.

Now I play memory games with myself. I'll try to recall something obscure. If I can't do it right away, I go about doing something else. Invariably the information I'm seeking suddenly pops into mind, just as it did that first time. Even though I now expect it, I'm still impressed when it happens.

Research on Stem Cell Therapy for Longevity

A study at the Duke University Medical Center, as published in Science magazine, had this to say:

Much of the increased risk for atherosclerosis progression with age may be a result of age-related declines in the capacity of precursor (stem) cells to repair damage in the arterial endothelium (artery wall)... Our study suggests that progenitor cell therapy might increase life expectancy in the population as much as the complete elimination of cancer.[xvi]

In the Proceedings of the National Academy of Sciences, a Stanford research team reported:

Def. *Aging results in a diminished capacity of the body to maintain tissue and organ function. Since we know the cells mediating this maintenance are stem cells, it doesn't take a leap of faith to think that (aging) stem cells are at the heart of that failure.[xvii]*

If this is the case, and I believe it is, what better source for maintenance of psychological and physiologic vitality than pristine fetal stem cells, resulting not only in longevity but in a far superior quality of life?

My patients commonly experience the benefits that I have reported in this chapter. They feel better, have more energy, and exhibit clearer, more efficient mental capacity. Medical tests we have conducted corroborate these findings, indicating that patients' physiological and cognitive biological markers score significantly younger than normal ranges for their chronological age.

For these benefits alone, I believe that fetal stem cell therapy should be widely available. Just imagine how much richer all of our lives would be if our elders remained healthier and alert throughout their later years, enjoying greater independence, fewer medical problems, and more able to contribute their knowledge, wisdom, and energy to society!

AIDS

According to the World Health Organization (WHO), 33 million people around the world are living with the AIDS virus. About 2 million die from AIDS each year, while another 3 million are newly infected. The WHO has declared the AIDS global epidemic to be the world's number one health threat.

There is currently no known cure for AIDS. It was originally thought that if the virus could be controlled at negligible levels, then that would affect a cure. Although treatment with a combination of anti-retroviral medications, such as AZT and other protease inhibitors, can reduce the HIV virus to a negligible level, a significant number of these patients eventually still develop the full spectrum of AIDS.

Scientists have now come to believe that the culprit lies in the strength of the immune system.

T-cells

AIDS is the acronym for "acquired immune deficiency syndrome." The disease kills by destroying the immune system. T-cells are the soldiers of your immune system. They recognize foreign invaders such as infections, and other threats, such as cancer. The human immunodeficiency virus (HIV) attacks and destroys T-cells, leaving the body defenseless against these foreign invaders.

To replicate, HIV must first enter the T-cell. Once it gets inside, the virus has the ability to commandeer the "control panel" of the T-cell, taking over its mechanisms and turning the once-beneficial, protective T-cell into a highly efficient, HIV-producing factory. Eventually, the infected T-cell virtually explodes, releasing copious amounts of newly created HIV, which then infect more T-cells, creating a geometric vicious cycle of HIV production.

As this process continues its deadly course, the body attempts to make up for the loss by producing new T-cells, but over time it is unable to keep up with their destruction by the HIV virus. The individual's immune system is first weakened and then eventually destroyed altogether.

The infections that are lying dormant in all of us, held down by our immune system, can then flourish unchallenged. . Thus allowing the ensuing opportunistic infections typical in AIDS victims, such as Kaposi's sarcoma (a form of cancer), pneumocystis pneumonia, and toxoplasmosis (a disease that damages the central nervous system) to thrive.

Unfortunately, the antiviral drugs presently used to treat HIV can cause a wide range of potentially dangerous side effects. Also, recent scientific evidence has shown that over time, HIV develops resistance to these drugs, making them less and less effective, sometimes even useless.

Ten years ago, I wondered if fetal stem cells could somehow interfere with the HIV'S deadly process. I began to develop a theoretical concept, and five years later I was fortunate to actualize the theory.

The CD4 Cell and CCR5 Co-receptors

Those infected with HIV may carry the virus for months or years and maintain a functioning immune system. But once their immune system weakens beyond a certain point, they will begin to manifest the previously described symptoms of AIDS.

The strength of our immune system can be measured in the laboratory by counting the number of a specific type of a T-cell called CD4.

✷A clinical indication that an HIV-positive person has made the transition to AIDS is a CD4 count of less than 200—normal being 550 to 1200.

In order for HIV to begin its destructive process, it must first gain entry into the CD4 cells by attaching itself to two co-receptors called CCR5, which provide a pathway for HIV to enter the CD4 cell. This means that, theoretically, an important research goal would be to find a method to prevent the HIV from using these CCR5 co-receptors to gain entry to the T-cells.

But where to begin?

It is known that some individuals seem to be naturally immune to HIV/AIDS. There are people who have engaged in unprotected sex with HIV-positive partners long-term without contracting the virus. And some children born to HIV-positive mothers are not infected.

Researchers discovered that the reason people in these two groups did not acquire AIDS was that due to a genetic mutation, they were missing both of the CCR5 co-receptors. Without that pathway for HIV to enter the CD4 cell, it couldn't infect them.

I reasoned that if we were able to isolate fetal stem cells from a fetus that was missing the CCR5 co-receptors, and then administer those cells to an HIV/AIDS patient, then fetal stem cell treatment might prove to be a major breakthrough in the treatment and even the prevention of AIDS.

The incidence of the CCR5 mutation is very rare, but eventually I was able to find a fetus that was missing the CCR5 co-receptors and isolate its stem cells.

I then administered these mutant fetal cells to an AIDS patient, Paul, who had been told by his doctor that nothing more could be done for him and that at best he had only a few weeks left to live.

When I met Paul, he could barely walk, even with assistance. Due to meningitis, he was profoundly confused and his speech was unintelligible. His CD4 count was 34, indicating that his immune system was essentially nonexistent.

After the fetal stem cell treatment, he began to show noticeable improvement almost immediately. Within two weeks, he was feeling significantly better; his mind was clear, and his CD4 count was rising dramatically, indicating the return of his immune system.

Two months after his treatment, all of the indicators of his immune status were within normal limits, and they have remained so ever since. Also, as one would expect, no opportunistic infections have returned.

Paul had only one fetal stem cell treatment and has been symptom-free for over four years. He reports that he has "never felt better," and that his mental acuity and energy are at higher levels now than before he became ill. He has regained his passion for living, including his interest in the study of languages. Today he is able to speak five languages, which he said he found "surprisingly easy to learn."

In addition to restoring his immunity and thereby freeing him from his death sentence, fetal stem cells provided Paul with all of the benefits that I discussed in the previous chapter.

Has Paul Been Cured? You decide

Experts will dismiss this successful case history on the grounds that it is an isolated event, an inexplicable "spontaneous recovery." They will suggest that to validate my treatment, I perform a large double-blind study wherein one group of AIDS patients receives the mutant fetal stem cells while the control group receives only a placebo.

As I have discussed throughout this book, I have a profound moral problem with that. I have seen this therapy work on Paul. If I were to conduct such a long-term double-blind study, ,required by "scientific method", I would be condemning the patients in the control group to needless further pain and suffering and eventually death—all to rule out the absurd possibility that my patients were being cured of AIDS by a placebo effect.

I became excited when I found two new recent articles regarding a possible treatment for HIV/AIDS. The first was in a British newspaper that described how a group of doctors had inadvertently discovered a method for treating AIDS that was similar to mine. They were treating their patient for Leukemia with a bone marrow transplant. In addition to leukemia, the patient also had HIV/AIDS. The article reported the patient was cured of the virus when doctors "exchanged his bone marrow with that of a donor with **a rare natural resistance to HIV (missing the CCR5)**."

161

As of the original publication of the research in *The New England Journal of Medicine* in February 2006, it had been three years since the procedure, and the man still showed no signs of the disease. According to the article, researchers are "confident the process will work for other sufferers," adding that it "could become common in just five years."

They said that they intended to conduct trials on additional AIDS patients and were hopeful that the therapy could be used to treat patients in the future. However, the potential for such bone marrow transplants in the treatment of AIDS *"is limited by the fact that besides the inherent difficulty in being able to find a matching donor, the odds of that donor also having the genetic mutation is minuscule."* "It won't be for everyone," one scientist said.[xviii]

Going back to my methodology, there is a challenge inherent in the procedure I used for my patient. It is estimated that only 1 to 3 percent of the general population is missing CCR5, which makes it difficult to obtain large quantities of these unique fetal stem cells. This is one of the main reasons that we have worked so hard to expand the number of stem cells that can be derived from a single fetus.

Scientists know how to grow fetal stem cells, but once the cells are expanded, they differentiate, meaning that they have become one of the 220 specific types of cells found in the human body and are no longer in their pluripotent state.

In contrast, our scientific team has developed a method whereby we are able to grow the fetal stem cells, successfully maintaining them in their pluripotent state. **One single fetus can now provide enough**

material to treat over a million patients, including those with HIV/AIDS.

I have also used a second successful method for treating AIDS. As you already have read, fetal stem cells significantly strengthen an individual's immune function. And since AIDS is a result of HIV suppressing and destroying immune function, I reasoned that normal, non-mutant fetal stem cells could keep the symptoms of AIDS under control by providing the patient with an entirely new, robust immune system.

Normal fetal stem cells do not prevent HIV from entering, attacking, and destroying T-cells, but they do provide that second, stronger immune system. When treated with this protocol, our HIV/AIDS patient's immune system eventually becomes impaired again.

At this point, the patient once again can be given the normal, non- mutated fetal stem cells. This protocol can be repeated as many times as required.

Ron was my first HIV/AIDS patient. I first treated him eight years ago by the method I have just described. Unlike the millions of other HIV/AIDS victims, Ron is in the unique position of being able to return to our clinic for more fetal stem cells whenever his CD4 count starts to significantly drop. The treatment immediately begins to reverse the CD4 decline, bringing it back to normal levels. Over the years, his visits to the clinic have become less and less frequent. My belief is that due to the fetal stem cells, his immune system is winning control over the virus.

Ron reports that all of his friends who contracted the HIV virus at the same time he did have since died. Today, Ron is a successful businessman, is active in sports, and continues to live a healthy and fulfilling life.

A recent study at UCLA's AIDS Institute consensually validated the approach of boosting the immune system by showing that two chemical compounds "may help the immune systems of HIV-infected persons fight the disease without invasive gene therapy." Researchers found that these compounds activate telomerase—the protein that boosts cells' ability to divide. The benefit is that immune cells keep dividing to producing new, robust cells that continue to destroy HIV-infected cells.[xix]

And yet, as mentioned before, fetal stem cells contain complete telomeres and activate the enzyme telomerase. It is not necessary to develop new drugs; we need to accept fetal stem cell therapy.

HIV/AIDS treatment today consists of using antiretroviral drugs such as AZT to combat the HIV virus. But these drugs, which initially worked so well, *are now starting not to work* because the virus is mutating into drug resistant forms.

Drug-resistant HIV is now emerging to a level of serious concern, according to The World Health Organization (WHO).

Studies published in AIDS, the official journal of the International AIDS Society, report that ten years ago, between 1 and 5 percent of HIV patients worldwide had drug-resistant strains. Now, it averages as high as 30 percent of new patients who are already resistant to the drugs.

In some high-risk populations' in the world, HIV drug resistance rates soar as high as 80 percent.

Adding to the problem; each year new drug resistant strains are being detected. There were 80 different documented strains in 2007 and then 93 in 2008, according to Stanford University's HIV Drug Resistance Database.

Dr. John Mellors, an HIV drug resistance expert at the University of Pittsburgh, recently stated, "People tend to be naive and optimistic that the boogie man's not going to come. It's coming. This virus is no different than any other pathogen throughout history that we've chased with antimicrobials, and it's always going to keep one step ahead of us."

What Dr. Mellors meant by keeping "one step ahead of us" is that by using antiviral medications, no matter what new drugs we discover, the HIV virus will eventually mutate into a drug resistant form, making the new medication ineffectual.

There is a major difference in mechanism and outcome between the treatment methodology currently being used today and what I advocate. The success of my HIV/AIDS treatment is not affected by a mutation of the virus, because unlike antiretroviral drugs that attack the virus, my method prevents the HIV virus—mutated or not—from attacking the immune cell by eliminating the pathway the virus uses to enter the cell.

Therefore, does this new approach now constitute a cure for AIDS?

According to the World Health Organization, about 2.5 million children under the age of 15 have AIDS worldwide, and somewhere in the world a child becomes orphaned every 14 seconds because his or her parents died of AIDS. Think of the enormity of that statistic. It equates to more than 250 new orphans each and every hour of the day and night.

AIDS got a head start on the world when our government and others paid little or no attention to its outbreak. We cannot continue to turn away from those who suffer.

The potential for fetal stem cell therapy to free millions from the devastating symptoms of AIDS needs to be studied and exploited now.

Alzheimer's Disease

The brain is the human body's most complex organ. It controls functions *Brain*
that affect all aspects of our lives: thoughts, emotions, speech,
movements, the senses, and involuntary body functions.

The brain's management of these functions depends on its
communications network, which is made up of billions of neurons, or
nerve cells. These cells send electrical messages to one another across
gaps called synapses. This allows information and instructions to be
processed by various parts of the brain, which are then relayed to various
organ systems.

Alzheimer's, a disease that affects 4.5 million men and women
in the United States, is a result of abnormal changes within these nerve
structures, causing communication pathways or bridges to break down
and eventually become permanently disconnected. Consequently, aspects
of brain functions that control memory, behavior, personality, and
various bodily functions can be lost. That's why Alzheimer's patients
can forget information and behavioral patterns that used to be second
nature—how to drive, how to behave in public, even how to get dressed.
One of the most devastating aspects of Alzheimer's is that patients, while
still appearing to be normal, lose the ability to recognize even their own
children or life partners.

Alzheimer's affects up to 50 percent of people older than 85.
Age increases the risk. For every five-year age group beyond 65, the
percentage of people with Alzheimer's doubles.

Alzheimer's disease has no known cure. Despite the call for
research into embryonic and fetal stem cell therapy as a potential

intervention for Alzheimer's disease by many—including the family of late President Ronald Reagan, who suffered for more than a decade before his death—mainstream researchers remain unconvinced that it's a promising therapy.

One leading stem cell research scientist stated that due to the inherent nature of the disease, we'll never be able to help an Alzheimer's patient with embryonic or fetal stem cells.

Nothing has ever been published to support his statement. It is merely the doctor's opinion—and it's wrong. Statements such as this, however sincere and well-intentioned, are part of the culture of inertia that blocks further exploration into the benefits that fetal stem cells can provide an Alzheimer's patient.

I have administered fetal stem cells to a number of patients who had early stage Alzheimer's disease. Here are three case histories.

Carl

Carl was the former dean of a prestigious graduate school, a well-known and respected teacher who had lectured around the world and written many books. Before I met Carl, he had over the past several months started to feel his mind "slowly slipping away," as he put it. Eventually, even finding his way home from his office became difficult.

Diagnosed with Alzheimer's disease, Carl became anxious and depressed. He was particularly worried about a major lecture he was to deliver before a large distinguished audience; he feared losing his train of thought and forget what he was about to say. For a man who had been celebrated all of his life for his academic brilliance and genius IQ, his Alzheimer's' symptoms became overwhelming.

When he contacted me, Carl said frankly that he was very skeptical that fetal stem cells could benefit him. We had several conversations in which he and primarily his wife asked many intense and pointed questions. In the end, they decided to proceed with treatment.

On the day of the procedure, I told him about the increase in cognitive function and creativity I'd noted in all my patients after receiving the cells, regardless of the primary condition afflicting them. I even mentioned the possibility of him saying something in his lecture and then thinking, "I didn't know that." He looked at me skeptically and dismissed the notion.

A week after his treatment, Carl called to say that he wasn't noticing any improvement and was going to cancel his lecture, which was six weeks away. I asked him to take it a day at a time and wait a few weeks before canceling. He reluctantly agreed. About two weeks later, Carl phoned me again, telling me that cognitive changes were becoming apparent, so for now he had decided to hold off on canceling his lecture. I did not hear from him again until the day after his presentation.

"Remember what you told me about what I might experience as I lectured?" He laughed. "Well, I found myself thinking that I wished I was in the audience, so I could take notes on what I was saying."

Carl opted for a second treatment six months after the first because, as he put it, "I'm doing so well, I want to insure that the process continues."

It has been over five years since Carl was first treated. To date he has no symptoms of Alzheimer's. He told me that he thinks that his mind is actually clearer today than it was years ago, and that he requires less sleep, gets up early, and attacks his writing with a new creative energy.

He wrote a letter to his doctor, giving him a progress report, and copied me:

As your patient, I wanted to give you an update on my progress. Subjectively, I think I am at the top of my form. Though I am semi-retired, I have been invited to continue to work with our international programs.

I am teaching a course with an eminent international scholar, and am about to begin to direct a program for continuing education for the graduate school. The new dean has asked me to teach a course with him next year, and I have been named Dean Emeritus, a title never before awarded at our graduate school.

I know that you are skeptical about my fetal stem cell treatment. I think you know that I try to remain scientific about truth. Indeed I completely and truly believe in the process.

My performance continues to be so greatly improved over that dark, pre–fetal stem cell period.

Don

Five months after receiving fetal stem cells, Don's wife wrote to me, describing the history of her husband's Alzheimer's disease.

Before Don received the fetal stem cells, his first signs of Alzheimer's were forgetfulness and difficulty following conversations. It then progressed to the point where sometimes he would get lost when going somewhere he'd been a hundred times. We even stopped going to the movies because he had a hard time following the plots.

We went on a previously planned cruise to Alaska, and most of the time he couldn't remember what we had done the day before. He would ask four or five times what we were doing next...he couldn't remember the names of the passengers we ate with every day.

Life at home was not good. It was difficult to talk to him about the simplest of things. He didn't make sense a lot of the time and he would stare off into space as if he wasn't there. Our world was getting smaller and smaller.

Don also had a personality change. He would get agitated and angry over things that had never bothered him before. He would yell and rant, and then sulk. All of this was new behavior. This was not the Don I knew.

On my doctor's suggestion, I went to an Alzheimer's caregivers support group. There it all suddenly made sense to me. They all had similar stories. They understood and had been through exactly the same life story I was living. It really upset me when they told me I should start researching to find a home to place him in. They told me that nothing could stop the decline, and it would happen very fast.

Then Don received the fetal stem cells. Four months later, the miracle began to happen. We were able to talk to each other again, and he was making sense. We spent a Sunday morning taking an IQ test just for fun on the computer, and he got almost all the answers right.

Was my old Don back? I was getting hopeful, but I expected he would backslide during a previously scheduled trip we were taking to Ireland. Well, we have just returned after three weeks traveling. Don did great on the trip. He continues to get better every day.

By William C. Rader, MD

I believe that stem cell treatment cured Don's Alzheimer's. To me, this is a miracle—a miracle that so many are looking for.

We found the fetal stem cells at just the right moment. And we are very grateful.

Jim

When Jim first came to me for treatment, his wife told me that before he developed Alzheimer's, they had an ideal marriage. She said she was very concerned by his sudden and severe deterioration and exhausted by having to manage every aspect of both their lives.

A month after Jim's treatment, she called me up and reported, "I definitely do like the positive changes I see in my husband, but now he's becoming a bit obstreperous because he is uncomfortable and resentful of my stronger position in our relationship."

I explained to her that because of his diminished mental capacity prior to treatment, Jim had no awareness of their role reversal, but now that his mind was clearing, he was cognizant of the change in their relationship. I suggested that she should, as much as possible, attempt to bring things back to normal.

A few weeks later, she called for advice, telling me that Jim was annoyed because everyone was telling him "how much he's changed for the better and that his mind is so much clearer. They keep telling him it's amazing, and he keeps insisting that his mind hasn't changed at all. It's really upsetting him."

I told her that even though these comments were obviously well intentioned, as far as Jim was concerned his mind had always been clear, and he clearly disliked being told otherwise.

If you break your arm, how do you know it's broken? Your mind tells you. If your mind is broken, you have no other internal means of evaluating your condition. The fetal stem cells can create such a positive cognitive change in an Alzheimer's patient that others immediately notice the difference. But Jim, who couldn't objectively observe what he was going through, could not perceive that anything had changed.

I then suggested to his wife that she explain this to their friends and family and ask them to please refrain from commenting on Jim's recovery.

Alzheimer's and the Immune System

A UCLA study, published in the *Journal of Alzheimer's Disease*, discovered that a deficiency in the immune system due to aging could lead to Alzheimer's disease by allowing plaques to accumulate in the brain—the hallmark of Alzheimer's disease. The body's immune system defends the brain from aging by cleaning the brain of these amyloid-beta waste products. A weakened immune system can cause an inability to "clean up" these plaque-forming waste products, resulting in Alzheimer's.[xx]

As I've noted, fetal stem cells strengthen the immune system at least tenfold; the cells also create new neural path-ways. Therefore, there are obvious advantages in using fetal stem cells as a treatment modality for both the prevention and treatment of Alzheimer's disease

Clearly each patient is different. By no means would I say that fetal stem cells are a cure for Alzheimer's. But I will say this:

By William C. Rader, MD

Nothing else known to medicine today can equal the level of positive outcome achieved with the clinical use of fetal stem cells in Alzheimer's patients.

I hope that one day soon, this new found awareness will stimulate an appropriate scientific inquiry, so that this therapy might relieve the suffering of millions of Alzheimer's patients, along with their families, that are now forced to watch helplessly as their loved ones decline and then eventually disappear.

Autism

Autism is the most widely diagnosed developmental disability in the United States, *affecting 1 in 110 children*, a dramatic rise from only a few decades ago, when the disease struck only *one out of every 10,000 children*. Removing factors such as more awareness of autism and therefore increased diagnosis, the figures still remain startling.

There are presently 1.7 million people living with autism, and an additional 24,000 children will be diagnosed this year alone. The Centers for Disease Control and Prevention (CDC) has labeled autism "an urgent public health concern."

Autism is characterized by withdrawal and an inability to communicate normally. Children with autism can also display severe compulsive behaviors, such as rocking, arm flapping, or repeated banging on objects, as well as ritualistic speech patterns. Autistic children diligently avoid eye contact. They can also engage in violent and self-destructive behavior, and they are prone to becoming epileptic.

No single cause has been attributed to autism, but some of the causative factors that have been linked to it are metabolic disorders, fetal *Causes* alcohol syndrome, abnormally small brain stem, heavy-metal poisoning, impaired or abnormal blood flow to the brain, viral infections, food allergies, adverse reactions to antibiotics, and defects in the myelinization process (the formation of the insulation of the body's nerve fibers).

Infant vaccinations have also been linked to autism, especially those including Thimerosol, a mercury containing product that was used solely as a preservative. (After some foot-dragging, and pressure from

Congress, vaccine manufacturers finally distributed a mercury-free version).

Autism has no known cure. Conventional medicine offers only symptomatic relief in the form of medications, usually antidepressants or drugs such as fenfluramine and haloperidol, to manage disruptive behavior. Such drugs can cause serious side effects and usually are recommended to be administered over the autistic person's entire life.

Sometimes improvements can be achieved when autistic children receive intensive cognitive and behavioral modification training and are placed on a regimen of healthy foods and nutritional supplements. However, no known treatment available today can equal the rapid, significant, and long-lasting improvements achieved by fetal stem cells.

I've treated many autistic children using fetal stem cell therapy, and they have consistently demonstrated remarkable improvements. Because they tend to be uncommunicative, many autistic children are assumed to have low IQ levels and are often labeled mentally retarded. I have found that these children generally have high IQs. After receiving fetal stem cells, these children move very quickly along the scale of maturation, being very proud of themselves as they readily master new skills.

After treatment, I encourage the children's parents to up the ante, so to speak, by raising expectations of them. Since the children know that their parents love them and would not ask them to do something they weren't able to, they gradually learn that they are now capable of new behaviors and achievements. Such parental reinforcement encourages them to fulfill their new, ever-expanding potential.

The following case histories include progress reports written by the autistic children's parents, who are the ones most capable of determining when and to what extent positive changes have occurred after treatment.

Before choosing fetal stem cell treatment for their children, almost all of the parents had tried every option available in conventional and alternative medicine, including cognitive and behavioral training. Without exception, they are loving, dedicated parents who have tirelessly educated themselves in their unrelenting quest to find help for their children. They are much like the real-life parents whose story was dramatized in the movie Lorenzo's Oil, who on their own created an original treatment for their child that is used to this day by the medical profession.

Many of these parents have been described, both privately and publicly, as taking "desperate measures." Actually, their choices are far from desperate. Quite the opposite: Their decisions are well thought-out and extensively researched. I spend many hours taking calls from parents who ask smart and appropriate questions, before choosing to proceed with fetal stem cell treatment.

None of the children presented in the following case histories had experienced any significant improvement from the treatments the parents had tried, other than the fetal stem cells.

Kyle

Dear Dr. Rader,

By William C. Rader, MD

I wanted to let you know about the amazing progress that my 5 year old son Kyle has made since entering into your care and receiving his stem cell transplant four months ago.

Kyle was evaluated by the Regional Center and given a diagnosis of mild to moderate Autism at age 3. We were devastated by the diagnosis and immediately began trying every therapy that could possibly help him. Most were ineffective or helped him only marginally.

Auditory processing was a huge problem for him. For years, Kyle would stare out the window of the car and could not hear us yelling his name. He was lost in his own world, and we struggled to break through to our son.

Before the stem cell treatment, Kyle had several issues we were dealing with. He was extremely hyperactive; spoke in short, scrambled sentences; sought pressure often, and had a very short attention span. He was placed in a special education kindergarten class, where he was the lowest functioning child in the room. Before the stem cells, the results of a blood test showed that his immune cells were very low, and that he was high risk for the H1N1 flu. His pediatrician said because of his weak immune system that Kyle was the type of child that could potentially die from contracting this virus—terrifying news for any parent to hear.

Now the good news—Two months after the stem cells treatment, his immune cell test had raised dramatically up to a normal level. And Kyle did contract the swine flu—and breezed through it with ease.

Shortly after receiving the stem cells, Kyle's speech patterns improved dramatically. Before the treatment, he uttered short sentences like "Where you go to go?" Now he is speaking in much longer and complete sentences. Everyone has commented that he is talking so much

178

more, and with greater clarity and purpose. For the first time in his young life, he is noticing the people and the world around him and taking it upon himself to interact with his surroundings. The last four months have been the most joyous of his young life!

Kyle used to be almost unable to sit at the dinner table, attend to any task, play a game, or show interest as a story was read to him. Today, he is like a different child altogether. He pays attention, makes comments, has many stories memorized and asks for more daily.

His interaction with friends and his little sister has greatly improved. Kyle is actually initiating and carrying on real conversations with us--recently he told me that Orion's Belt is his favorite constellation! He now thrills us with tales of some day taking driving lessons so he can use our car!

Due to this miraculous improvement, Kyle was quickly moved out of his special ed class and into a mainstream kindergarten class. We are over the moon with this latest development! I'm including the report that I just received, this report is from the Behavior Therapy Supervisor.

"On greeting Kyle, he looked me directly in the eye and said "Hi", using my name. In the two previous years of observation, he had never done this. Watching him sit and do a task in a kindergarten classroom was incredible, given several months before he was sitting in a large bucket of blocks, placing block after block on top of his legs and body to meet his sensory needs. In the span of 4 months, Kyle is now in the regular education classroom and has already surpassed his year-end educational/behavioral goals. It has been both exciting and an honor bearing witness to the changes this child has made in such a short period of time."

One specific instance shines a light for us on Kyle's progress. Over the past few years, we have attended his holiday pageant at school. To see that he was the only child in the school that had to be held on a teacher's lap was devastating to us. But last week, Kyle received an award for being the most well behaved, responsible and safe child in his normal kindergarten class. He heard his name called, walked up to shake the principal's hand, and stood proudly with the other children on stage. He held his certificate up high with a big smile. We were so proud of him, and so grateful for the moment. Later, the assistant principal called and asked bluntly, "What are you doing with Kyle? I can't believe the changes in him!"

And the wonderful moments have kept coming. Recently, we lay in our backyard hammock together, and Kyle pretended it was a pirate ship and I was the captain. We sailed the high sea and searched for treasures. He was calm, focused and present. It was just so normal!

Overall, Kyle is now doing amazingly well. He is the ringleader to his little friends, and goes out of his way to meet and engage new kids. He is very polite, shares with others and takes turns. Academically, he is now right on track for his age. He is such a great little guy.

We fervently believe that the stem cells treatment from you Dr. Rader has given us our wonderful, extremely charming, funny, empathetic, social, engaging and loving child.

Evelyn

Evelyn was eight years old when her parents brought her for treatment. When we met, she was completely uncommunicative. She ran around the room in circles, screaming and touching everything in sight.

She did not respond to any verbal suggestions or even commands from her parents. Her mother told me that aside from restraining her physically, controlling her was almost impossible.

Within weeks after receiving the fetal stem cells, Evelyn's behavior started to normalize. Very slowly at first, but as the months and years passed, she improved to the point that she could attend a regular school. Her mother kept me posted as to her progress on a regular basis.

The following is a letter I received from her mother, three years after her initial treatment.

Today Evelyn went to class and remembered that she had been working on a picture of a bowl of fruit, but her teacher had forgotten that and instructed her to start a picture of a doll instead. Unable to convince the teacher, and being clear and determined, Evelyn decided to continue drawing a bowl of fruit. Later, her teacher realized her error and told Evelyn that she was right (Great teacher).

Also, she has taken a liking to basketball and is making baskets from different areas of the court. She seems to love the sport. She also loves to ride her bike and to skate.

Evelyn is able to sit perfectly still in the dentist's chair when work is being done. Her dentist is amazed at how well she behaves. I forgot her dental appointment this morning and Evelyn cried, because she remembered it and wanted to keep her appointment (To see a dentist!)

More and more, she is able to make associations about technical subjects, even diabetes. She has a friend named Freddy who has diabetes. One day Freddy's finger was bandaged after having blood drawn. "What happened to Freddy's finger?" Evelyn asked. I told her that blood was drawn to test Freddy's blood sugar. When I told her that Freddy had diabetes and had to have a blood test to make sure he was okay, Evelyn wanted to know all about diabetes and how blood sugar levels relate to it.

On another occasion, as we enjoyed the story of The Hunchback of Notre Dame together, Evelyn became absorbed in trying to figure everything out. What was Esmeralda's relationship with the hunchback and Silvio? Why were they going to burn Esmeralda at the stake? She wanted to know everything. When I hesitated to remember the answer to her questions, she smiled, making her eyes sparkle. Then she laughed, just as she laughs at me when she whistles, because I can't whistle.

Today I brought Evelyn with me when I was getting my hair done. She sat in the waiting room calmly until I was finished, something that obviously would not have been even close to possible before. When I was finished and returned to the waiting room, she looked up at me, smiled, and said, "Cool haircut."

When we returned home, I told her to take a shower. At first she didn't pay attention to me, humming to herself as she lay on her bed reading a book. I fully expected her to be doing the same thing when I returned to her room. But when I got upstairs, much to my surprise I found her in the bathroom in the shower and washing herself. When I pulled back the shower curtain, Evelyn, teasing me, gave me a knowing grin.

What I am most impressed about my wonderful Evelyn is that she often asks me, "When are we going back to see Dr. Rader? I want to get even better."

Carl

    Carl is another autistic child who greatly benefited from fetal stem cell treatment. What follows is Carl's story, told in his mother's own words from letters she wrote me after I treated Carl.

When Carl was born he came quickly and was of normal, average weight. He seemed like a typical baby boy. At five weeks of age, Carl had a fever of 105 degrees. The pediatrician sent us directly to the hospital, where we stayed for three days. Carl was given antibiotics, both by IV and by spinal tap. A few weeks after Carl was released from the hospital, at the urging of the pediatrician, he received a vaccination cocktail (multiple vaccines administered together in a single injection). He had an immediate and continued severe negative reaction.

For the first three months after the vaccination, he cried fiercely and often. Unable to sleep, he would cry regularly from 10 p.m. until 3 a.m. At five months, he was able to fall asleep in my arms while I rocked him, and I would put him in his crib; but he would wake later and I would have to bring him to bed with me.

During the day I would drive him around in the car, and it would calm him down and he would act fine until I came to a stoplight. Then he would begin to cry again, and when we started moving again his crying would become so intense, it became almost impossible for me to concentrate on my driving.

Carl's physical development seemed normal. He crawled and then walked in a timely fashion. Later, Carl engaged in hugging, but the way he squeezed people, it seemed more like a way of flexing his muscles. Although he related to some extent to his environment, his way of doing so was not at all like his sister, who is just 16 months his senior.

Carl was 18 months old when a major negative change occurred. It was like the light went out and Carl was gone. He didn't make any more sounds, and he didn't look at objects or make eye contact with anyone. Instead he would just inappropriately clap his hands, walk about on his toes, and wander away from any social situation.

At that time, we had several special education teachers whom we knew, and I asked them if they would personally observe Carl. They called me back within a few days after seeing him, with an extremely negative report; Carl was severely autistic. I was devastated and bewildered about how to proceed.

One night I hugged Carl and made a solemn promise to him and myself that no matter what it took I was going to bring him back. Carl didn't resist my hug, but he didn't really respond to it, either, and then he just walked away.

My husband was in denial; he had a hard time believing anything was wrong with his child. He basically left me to take care of Carl. My marriage would end two years later.

I tried anything and everything that made sense to help Carl. Nothing seemed to work. It was very depressing. I used a special home-school program for a year, while I was working full time. The instructors would close him away in a room so that he wouldn't be "distracted" while they worked with him. The reality was that they didn't want anyone to see what they were doing. I later learned, after I requested Carl's file, that for an entire year the instructors tried consistently to get Carl to answer the same question correctly ten times in a row. Even when Carl was able to answer it nine times, they refused to move on. When I questioned them about this, they told me that Carl was stubborn, as if he had to be broken like a horse.

Once Carl was old enough, he began attending a special school with more open-minded teachers who were specifically trained to deal with autistic children. With their help over a number of years, Carl became slightly more verbal. But then he started to lose ground again.

This was Carl's condition when his mother brought him to me for treatment. Three months after he received fetal stem cells, his mother wrote me the following progress report:

I have noticed positive changes in Carl both specific and general. His therapist, aides, and teacher have all commented on his improvement.

I have not told them about the fetal stem cell treatment, because I didn't want them looking for anything negative to happen. They report that Carl is calmer, more focused, more easily engaged, and much happier. He now responds to praise and understands what it means. Everyone who spends any time with him comments that Carl is now able to understand everything they say. He is also much more responsive to complex demands. Before, if I asked him to go upstairs to put his clothes on, I used to have at best one chance in twenty that he would comply. Now the odds are more like one in four.

Carl is also much more easily redirected, and I am able to discern what is bothering him when he is upset. He also calms down much more quickly when he is taken care of, and I can actually reason *with him. If we're driving and I turn in a direction other than what he expects, he may protest for a moment, but he responds well to my explanation and then accepts it. Before, when I tried to explain things to him, it made no difference. He would just continue to act out and cry.*

He is also continuing to speak spontaneously, without coaxing. This has definitely improved over the last three months. He's saying many words and has a good amount of recall of words without prompts. When I say, "Good night, Carl," he replies, "Good night, Mommy," instead of robotically repeating, "Good night, Carl," the way he used to do. This continues to be a big thrill for me.

Carl has also been making more of a definite attempt to communicate in order to get what he wants. Recently he had a fit, so I put him in his room. I stood at the bottom of the stairs, and he kept coming out into the hall. I pointed to his door and told him to go back in and shut the door. He complied, but only for a few seconds. We repeated this two more times. Then I told him he couldn't come out unless he calmed down and stopped yelling. With that, he said, "Okay," and started coming down the stairs. I nearly died, because we had never had such an interaction, and especially not such a casual positive response from him.

Another improvement has to do with Carl's television viewing. Previously he would torture us by watching the same movies and videos over and over, day after day. Now he's happy to watch a variety of things with us. He also used to continually take off his shoes in and out of the house, in the car, in the store—everywhere! Now, if I tell him to keep his shoes on, he will. He has grown much taller and is able to walk flat-footed, instead of how he used to always walk on his toes.

I cannot express what it means to me to have fulfilled the promise I made to Carl and myself, that fateful day, after being told all hope was lost.

Margaret

Margaret is another of my patients. She attended a special Montessori school for children with autism and other cognitive disabilities. Margaret's condition was so severe that neither her parents nor her teachers knew for sure if Margaret was even aware that she was in classroom with other children. She made no eye contact with anyone, just sat listlessly at her desk or acted out with inappropriate behavior.

Her mother wrote:

"Despite countless hours of educational therapy and biomedical intervention in an attempt to get my daughter to express any type of language skills, there was zero improvement. Margret's learning basically did not improve at all for about five years".

This went on from the time Margaret was three years old until she turned eight, when her parents brought her to me.

A few days after her first fetal stem cell treatment, Margaret began to utter a few phrases. A number of weeks later, her teacher phoned Margaret's mother and was in tears because of how excited she was. That day, Margaret had stood up from her desk to walk over to each child in her class. She greeted each one of them by name, saying, "Hi, my name is Margaret."

By William C. Rader, MD

Margaret then went up to her teacher and introduced herself, also greeting her by name. Her teacher was astonished. Until that moment, the teacher and Margaret's parents were convinced that she had no awareness of anyone else in the classroom, let alone their names. Her teacher said the other children were "ecstatic." She then told Margaret's mother, "This has been the most promising, wonderful day that I've had in six years!" Since that day, Margaret plays with and relates to her classmates like any normal child.

In a follow-up letter to me relating Margaret's progress, her mother writes:

Today Margaret took her teacher's hand and turned to her classmates. "Let's go, guys," she said, and began to lead her teacher toward the door to the playground. Her teacher allowed her to do so in order to see what Margaret was going to do. At the door, Margaret looked up at her and said, "I just wish I could pick my favorite friends and tell them, 'Let's go out and play!'"

Margaret is now soaking up knowledge like a sponge. The fact that she can now sit with her classmates and take spelling tests with her own list of words is like a miracle. Her teacher had tried to teach Margaret to write and spell for five years without any success. Now she scores 100 on almost every spelling test!

Equally dramatic is the improvement in Margaret's social skills. She has begun to "hang out" with her favorite girlfriends from school, and has been invited to a number of birthday parties and two social outings—one to the mall and the other to go swimming. This would have been unthinkable before her stem cell treatment.

Two years later, when Margaret turned ten, her mother wrote me another progress report. Margaret and her family had gone to a resort for a vacation.

We were dining and I arranged for Margaret to sit either at my table or to sit with her teenaged brother and his friends. To my surprise, Margaret decided she was going to sit at the table with the girls her age. She walked across the crowded dining room and sat and ate like a little lady, without supervision. I don't think I was ever as proud of her as I was at that moment!

Just for you to understand the full significance of this, I should add that many of the women I have befriended who have children with autism have told me that they have become increasingly isolated over the years, unable to socialize due to their children's behavior in public.

Finally, I want to add that Margaret is now showing that she feels hurt when she has done something to displease me, and showing great pride and happiness when she does something that I compliment her on.

I can truthfully say that because of my daughter's stem cell treatment, she has come out of her own world to be an active, loving participant in ours.

William

Unlike Margaret, who was severely withdrawn before her treatment, William was extremely hyperactive and prone to violence. Because of his behavioral problems, William was a full-time student at what is known as a discreet trial method school.

By William C. Rader, MD

William first received the fetal stem cells when he was five years old. In a follow up report, his father wrote:

Before William received the fetal stem cells, he was assaulting his teachers an average of five times per day. His violent behavior prompted the school, in conjunction with state law, to initiate an assault class that required all the teachers to attend special training, so that they would be better able to handle him.

Immediately after William's stem cell treatment, his assaults against his teachers were reduced to zero, and this continues to this day. It was a happy day for us when the school, a few weeks after William's return from treatment, ripped up the assault plan.

Before the stem cell treatment, we were reluctantly but strongly considering placing William in a full-time residential center, because of how uncontrollable he was. Now there is a calm that has come over him. In fact, this summer, almost every weekend, boys William's age came up to him and asked him to play with them. Before, they would have been afraid to do so.

When he does something, William is eager to share his accomplishments with his us, happily asking, "Mommy, Daddy, did you see what I did?"

On one occasion, he told me that he did not want to be disturbed because he was fully absorbed in a game. Remember, before, he was always agitated and unable to concentrate on anything.

Since the stem cells, he has quickly developed computer skills. In addition, he is now proving to be very good in academics, especially mathematics.

One time, at the dinner table, I was attempting to correct William's brother's mispronunciation of the word "spaghetti." His brother was not listening, apparently more interested in eating the spaghetti than pronouncing it correctly, causing me to say it again. William got up from his chair and walked over to me and said, "Dad, cut it out. He's trying to eat." My wife and I began to laugh, because for us, such a demonstration of clear communication and understanding was such a stark contrast to what we had experienced in the past with William. It was incredibly wonderful.

Today he surprised me at the local deli by greeting the owner by name. I still have no idea how he learned the man's name. When we went to the bank, he went over to a woman who works at a desk in the main area. William had not seen her in a few months, but he still said hi to her, greeted her by name, and introduced his brother to her.

Whenever someone new is introduced to him, he says, "Hi, my name is William." He's always bringing a smile to people's faces when we go out, and he now knows how cute he is. When I call home, he asks Mom to let him talk to me, and he can answer questions about how his day went. Previously, when he got on the phone he would just talk gibberish and not listen to the other person. Now it's a conversation.

William is now even better behaved than his normal brothers, and when they go on trips together he is able to sit calmly in his seat at the airport whereas before he could not do so at all.

I witnessed this firsthand when I was at the airport with William and his father on the way to the clinic for William's first fetal stem cell treatment. He refused to sit down and instead would walk all about, jumping up and down on every empty seat, requiring his father to follow him all around the airport. Despite the angry and judgmental stares from other travelers, William's father was very patient and never scolded him because he knew that William was incapable of behaving any better because of his autism. (What a great parent!)

In one of his letters, William's father enclosed a chart related to William's progress since receiving fetal stem cells. The chart is known as the Assessment of Basic Language and Learning Skills (ABLLS).

Before beginning treatment, William was at 20 percent of normal skills, according to the ABLLS chart. A few months after the treatment, William's chart showed that he was at 85 percent of normal.

In another letter, William's father wrote:

William is happy all the time now and a joy to be around. When I come home from work, he greets me with a smile on his face and asks, "Daddy, did you have a good day?" I can't express in words what that means to me!

The other day William told his mother, "I want Daddy to be happy and proud." And I am happy and proud!

In a recent telephone conversation, William's father shared with me; that the entire family had recently gone to dinner at a restaurant. In the middle of dinner a complete stranger walked up to William and handed him a dollar, saying, *"Whenever I see a really well-behaved child I give them a dollar."*

Audrey

An important factor in recovery from autism is a behavioral change in the parents. Because of their long experience with the autistic behaviors of their child and the parents' inability to change them, the parents can feel stuck—unable to imagine ever having any significant control over their child's conduct.

When I meet with parents of autistic children, I carefully explain that their child, after receiving the fetal stem cells, may become more responsive and willing to comply with their requests, an important component in learning and growth. It usually takes several of these conversations before the parents can fully grasp this concept because they are naturally gun-shy after years of difficulty with their child.

Audrey's mother called me one day, very excited. She told me that although she had understood what I told her a few months back, she still feared being firm with her daughter. She told me that before her treatment, Audrey routinely exhibited difficult behavior whenever she rode in the car. As soon as she got into the car, Audrey would insist that music be played on the radio. When they arrived at their destination and the radio was shut off, Audrey would scream uncontrollably and refuse to leave the car. When Audrey was finally coaxed out of the car, she refused to close the car door.

That day, when Audrey and her mother got into the car, her mother turned on the radio, then turned to Audrey and said in a firm, clear tone, "When we stop the car, I am going to turn off the radio and you will not make a sound. Then you will get out of the car and close the door." When they reached their destination, Audrey's mother stopped the car and the shut off the radio. Her heart pounded as she waited to see what would happen. At first, Audrey was silent and sat still. Then, without further prompting, she opened the car door, got out, and closed the door. Audrey's mom now clearly understood the concept of higher expectations.

As autistic children begin recovery, they have no idea what their capacity for achievement is because they have been prevented by their disorder from discovering it. Therefore, it is critical to encourage parents to raise expectations and to communicate those expectations to their children in a loving way, with plenty of positive reinforcement for good behavior and achievement.

As the fetal stem cells continue their work, new connections are forged in autistic children's brains, enabling them to continue their cognitive growth. Also, every time they achieve something new, they are very proud of themselves, as well they should be. Each step they take toward normal behavior is a very significant achievement. Their parents tell me the smiles on their faces and the pride in what they are now able to accomplish is a true joy to behold.

Parents, who know far more about their autistic children than I or any other physician, scientist, or researcher ever will, report that their children continue to improve months, even years, after receiving fetal stem cells. I don't know how any scientific test or study could be more definitive.

Suzanne Wright, cofounder of Autism Speaks, a national clearinghouse for autism information, says, "Too many parents go to bed each night praying that one day their child will look them in the eye, smile, and say, 'Mommy.'" The prayers of the parents of the autistic children that you have just read about, as well as the many others whose children have received fetal stem cell treatment, are being answered.

Bell's Palsy

Bell's palsy is the most common cause of facial paralysis. It is a consequence of damage to one of the two facial nerves; with only one side of the face affected, the result is significant facial distortion.

Symptoms may include weakness or paralysis of one side of the face, drooping of an eyelid or a corner of the mouth, twitching, drooling, impairment of taste, and excessive tearing in the eye. Most scientists believe that a viral infection causes the disorder by creating an inflammation or swelling of the facial nerve, thereby rendering it inactive.

According to current medical wisdom, there is no known cure or standard course of treatment for Bell's palsy. The prognosis for most individuals with Bell's palsy is generally good, but in some cases the symptoms are permanent.

Maria is the only patient who has come to me requesting treatment for Bell's palsy. Three weeks after her fetal stem cell treatment, Maria wrote:

Dear Dr. Rader,

First of all I am writing to you to thank you, thank you, and thank you for having brought hope into my life.

Before my Bell's palsy, I kept my life very busy between my job, my family, and my personal life. Everything was fine. Then suddenly one day, for no reason, my body started shaking uncontrollably. I was taken to the hospital where over the next five days they gave me all the tests they could think of to find out what was wrong with me: a CAT scan, cardiogram, spinal tap, MRI and blood tests, including checking to see if I had a virus. After five painful days of testing and poking, nothing was found. I was sent home with a horrendous pain in my neck and shoulders, killing headaches, and Vicodin for all my pain. After that came the outpatient follow-ups. I was told that they were still unable to find a cause for my Bells Palsy and nothing more could be done for me.

All this was four years ago.

When I came to see you, half of my body, including my face, was paralyzed. I had been living with constant headaches and I had a continual drumming in my ear which was driving me crazy. My speech was slurred due to the left side of my mouth being paralyzed. I had joint pain, my left eye vision was blurry, and I was seeing double. I had constant sinus problems because of the pressure of my left nose muscle, which made it difficult to breathe. I had numbness and trembling in the entire left side of my body. I forgot things which I would have had no problem remembering before I became sick. Although I felt like a complete wreck, I would act happy at my job and around all the people that knew me, because I did not want anyone to feel sorry for me.

Today is three weeks and two days since my stem cell treatment, and I'm excited to tell you the results have been absolutely wonderful. My headaches are gone! The numbness and trembling in my leg has completely stopped, and my sinuses have cleared up so I can breathe easily. And I no longer have that continuous drumming in my ear! I can't begin to tell you what a relief that is.

I can see more clearly, and I have absolutely no pain in my joints. The muscles in my face are starting to move, so I'm looking much more normal. Also, my speech is improving every day, and now everyone can understand me better. When I look in the mirror now, I hardly recognize myself. I am starting to look like my old self.

I thank God first, and then I thank you, Dr. Rader, for your wisdom in utilizing your medical knowledge, your kindness, and your generosity for not charging me for my treatment.

You have given me the opportunity to be able to look up to my life and face the world.

For all of this I will be eternally grateful.

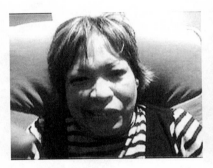

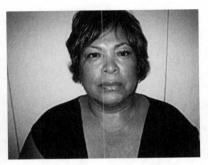

Maria on the day of treatment   *Maria five weeks later*

Brain Damage

The brain is our primary organ for coordinating and regulating all of the body's physiological activities and cognitive functions. It is composed of neurons (nerve cells) and neuroglia (supporting cells), housed within gray and white matter. The gray matter is composed primarily of nerve cell bodies. The white matter is composed of nerve cell processes that form tracts connecting various parts of the brain.

Think of the brain as the driver's seat of consciousness, thought, memory, reason, and judgment. It communicates with its nerve cells through a distinct group of chemicals known as neurotransmitters. Through the neurons and neuroglia, the brain sends and receives impulses, or messages, to and from the entire body. It directs the senses and the body's other systems—circulatory, cardiovascular, gastrointestinal, hormonal, motor, respiratory, and so on.

The brain requires a consistent blood flow to supply enough oxygen to satisfy the heavy metabolic demands of its neurons. Any decrease in blood flow can trigger a catastrophe because the brain is the organ most susceptible to a lack of oxygen. That catastrophe is what we call brain damage.

Brain damage can produce a wide range of devastating effects, including impaired functioning in one or more of the body's systems, difficulties in comprehension and learning, impaired memory, personality disorders, impaired speech, problems with balance and gait, partial or full paralysis, tremors, loss of control over bodily functions, and a host of other disabilities.

By William C. Rader, MD

There are various causes of brain damage, such as head trauma, complications at birth, stroke, brain lesions, allergic reactions, tumors, reactions to vaccines, and exposure to toxins. Whatever the cause, the result is the same: lack of oxygen to the sensitive neuronal cells. Conventional medicine often cannot provide more than minor relief and management of symptoms. By contrast, fetal stem cell therapy can provide positive results in the treatment of brain damage. That's because fetal stem cells can "wake up" dormant areas of the brain (cytokines) and then repair and replace damaged nerve cells. As the following examples demonstrate, fetal stem cell treatment addresses the damage itself–not merely the symptoms.

Here are six of my patients' case histories illustrating the power of fetal stem cells in reversing brain damage.

Gary

Gary was born a normal, healthy boy. Shortly after, tragedy struck. He suddenly began bleeding into his brain. By the time he was resuscitated, his brain had been without oxygen for about 30 minutes. Gary lapsed into a coma and was placed on life support.

His doctors declared that Gary was in a vegetative state. He was blind, could barely hold his head up, and his muscles were in spasm. He could produce no sound, express no emotion, or comprehend anything that was said to him. In short, Gary was incapable of any of the activities a normal infant could perform, including eating. A permanent feeding tube was surgically inserted though his abdomen directly into his stomach. He was even incapable of having bowel movements on his own.

Gary's doctors strongly recommended institutionalizing him. They said absolutely nothing could be done to improve his condition and that it would only get worse with time.

But his parents refused. They believed that, because of the level of care required for Gary, institutionalization would be tantamount to a death sentence.

When I first saw Gary, he was three years old and still in an unresponsive vegetative state. Three months after he received the fetal stem cells, his mother wrote me this report:

Gary is starting to make sounds! He is using tone and pitch to emphasize things. He is making "ga-ga" sounds and has added emphasis to his cooing sounds. Gary is now able to let us know when he is happy or unhappy, comfortable or uncomfortable, which allows us to know and respond to his needs.

He is also smiling, laughing, and overall is very happy. Previously he had no emotional reaction at all. Now he is showing a full range of emotions, and he has different facial expressions. This is incredible because at long last Gary is responding.

Gary is also using his eyes more. One of the therapists, who has worked for many years with numerous blind children, tells me that Gary is no longer acting like a blind child at all! Gary has also started burping and passing gas, neither of which he'd ever done before his stem cell treatment. This is an indication that his digestive tract is starting to work, which is another wonderful change.

Another noticeable improvement that began shortly after Gary received the stem cells is that he now has head control. Before, when I picked him up, if I forgot to cradle his head, it would just flop back. He is working so hard, and he's holding his head up for longer and longer periods of time, and is also able to move his head around more. If he needs to drop his head so he can rest, he's not allowing it to flop down the way it used to, but really making an attempt to control it.

All the therapists are excited to see such positive changes happening with Gary. Just as important, the stem cells seem to be helping each therapy session rapidly produce more and more positive results. Gary is also showing anticipation from verbal cues, another sign that he is now able to comprehend when he is being spoken to.

Now I love to cradle Gary in my arms, and ask him if he's ready to spin. Then I twirl him around in a circle a few times. Then we "unspin" by twirling in the opposite direction. He loves this! He laughs and kicks and moves his arms all over the place in glee, and often he squeals in delight. Whenever I ask him if he's ready to spin, he gets very excited, his eyes grow large, and he has a big smile on his face. Then he will start kicking his legs and make noise to indicate how excited he is. Because of this, I know Gary is now able to understand things that are about to happen in the future, instead of just responding to what is happening now.

When I make a sound to imitate laughing, Gary will smile and laugh back. This is so awesome to see and hear!

A few weeks later, Gary's mother wrote again:

Gary did something new last night. I was tickling him and he was laughing. I always tell him, "I am tickling you," as I'm tickling him, and I can get him to really giggle and belly laugh. But I would always have to tell him I was tickling him for this response to occur. Today, I told him, "I'm going to tickle you," and he started laughing with anticipation before I even touched him. This was a first.

The nurse, who assists us in Gary's care, seeing this, cried out in astonishment, "Did you see that? Gary is able to comprehend things." It left me weeping with tears running down my face.

Before he received the fetal stem cells, he would often go days without really sleeping, and when he was awake I had to always hold him. My husband and I are a real team when it comes to Gary's care, working in shifts. Before receiving the stem cells, Gary would not fall asleep until sometime between 1 and 4 a.m., and sometimes not until 6 or 7 a.m. When he did sleep, he would usually wake up one to five times. Sometimes he would remain awake for hours before finally falling back asleep again. I would stay up all night tending to him, trying to catch snatches of sleep while he was sleeping. Then my husband would get up at 7 to give Gary his medications and first feed before getting ready to go to work.

Since Gary received the stem cells, we all are able to go to sleep at the latest by 1 a.m. and are able to get an uninterrupted, good night's sleep. Now if Gary does wake up in the night, all I have to do is reposition him in bed and he falls right back to sleep.

This is a miracle! As a result, my husband and I are gaining back some of our once normal lives.

Gary received one fetal stem cell treatment per year over the next four years. His improvement was constant and dramatic. In her latest report, his mother wrote:

We took Gary to the doctor for evaluation. The results of a SPECT (single photon emission computed tomography) brain scan showed a significant improvement in blood flow and metabolism compared to prior scans.

All of the physicians who spoke with us about the results of the brain scan were baffled and unable to explain the dramatic repair of Gary's brain, which they said they had never seen or even read about before.

I don't think there is a day that I don't cry from joy over all the gains our son continues to make. We have a faith in God that has only been strengthened since our little boy was injured.

It is awesome to watch this God-given miracle in progress!

Louis

Louis was just 16 months old the night he became brain damaged. His parents put him to bed as they did every night, but sometime later Louis woke up and climbed out of his crib. He had never done this before, and his parents didn't know he was capable of it. He then crawled undetected through an open sliding door into the back yard and fell into the swimming pool.

Louis had stopped breathing by the time his parents discovered what had happened and pulled him out of the pool. Although his father resuscitated him by performing CPR, Louis's brain had been deprived of oxygen for such a long time that he was left, according to the doctors, in a permanent, severely brain-damaged state. He was completely unresponsive, unable to lift his head or control its movements, and could not chew or swallow food. He also developed scoliosis, a curvature of the spine.

A pump was surgically implanted in Louis to provide a constant release of Baclofen, which helps prevent severe muscle spasms. Excess fluids that collected in his trachea had to be suctioned frequently, because they made breathing difficult. This alone required constant supervision.

I first met Louis three and a half years after his accident. His parents considered fetal stem cells to be Louis's last hope since they had exhausted all traditional and alternative medical interventions they were able to find. As in Gary's case, they had been told that not only was there no hope for Louis's improvement, but that he would only get worse and ultimately die.

When his parents came to me, they feared that he would not live much longer. After Louis received the fetal stem cells, his mother wrote:

The changes in Louis have been miraculous. Here is a list of the progress we've seen in him since he was treated.

In general, Louis has become much more aware and is able to understand what is said to and asked of him. He anticipates activities when he is told what is going to happen, and for the first time in his life he has started to smile. Seeing that sweet smile brought tears to our eyes.

His breathing is much more normal. He breathes more deeply and without noise from the fluid buildup in his throat, and now rarely needs to be suctioned. He is also handling his secretions better by coughing up mucus. His reflexive pupil response to light is now perfect, whereas before his pupils were fixed and dilated.

He can now eat one full jar of baby food, he swallows more consistently, and he is finally able to close his mouth around a spoon. His bowel movements are much more regular as well.

He has much better head control now and is even able to hold his head up when he is carried. He is starting to move his left leg, and he is able to purposely grasp things with his left hand as well. His right hand, which had become rigid and closed, has now released.

In her next report, Louis's mother wrote:

Louis has remained very healthy, without any sign of infections. Before the stem cells, he would become sick very often. Another big development is that the Baclofen pump has been dramatically reduced without any return of his painful muscle spasms. He can now understand simple commands; as a result, he's become much more vocal. He laughs out loud, and his breathing is so much better that he can blow a horn.

He is beginning to be able to oppose his left index finger and thumb in a pincher grip. He's able to roll over from a supine position all by himself, and he gives me huge hugs. He now has the ability to understand complex commands and is displaying an increased range of emotions and is engaged socially He has more likes and dislikes and is able to express them. He is more interested in and aware of other children, and he is also developing a sense of humor.

The physical improvements are continuing, too. He is growing taller and gaining weight. In addition, his scoliosis has improved by 40 percent!

My son, who was supposed to remain emotionless and motionless, is now crawling around like crazy and is constantly happily laughing out loud.

As of today, Louis continues to make rapid improvement in physical and cognitive abilities and emotional and social responsiveness. The degree and rate of his improvement have never in the history of medicine been reported in a patient with such severe brain damage.

Lily

Lily suffered a stroke immediately after she was born. The resulting brain damage left her blind and deaf, she could not make any sounds, had little control over her body, and her head hung downward listlessly.

Lily's neurologist declared that she was in a vegetative state and recommended that she be institutionalized.

A little over three months after Lily received fetal stem cells, her mother wrote me this progress report:

A miracle occurred. From being deaf and blind, Lily is now able to see and hear! She has also begun to make sounds. Lily has a lot more control over her body now, which is especially noticeable in her head and her back. She is vocalizing a lot and beginning to make different sounds instead of only the vowel sounds that she began making soon after she received the cells. She is also starting to verbalize as we spend time with her using flashcards.

She is becoming more and more alert with each passing day and has a new curiosity about life, reaching out to touch things that she is now able to see for the first time. I am always noticing new positive changes in her.

Her understanding is coming right along, and she will look at you when you call her name. You have to understand that after being told our beautiful little child would always be a "vegetable," seeing her do something new every day is like a little chunk of heaven!

Brandon

Brandon suffered a freak accident while competing in a college track meet. For safety's sake, javelin and discus events aren't typically conducted while races are being run. But just as Brandon's race started, a discus thrower decided to get in some practice. His throw struck Brandon squarely in the forehead.

As a result of his injury, Brandon was in a coma for about three and a half weeks. In his own words, Brandon recalls the following:

When I woke up, I had no use of my legs and my right arm, was unable to speak, and had to learn everything all over again because I had no memory of my life before the accident.

Though he eventually regained use of his extremities and some of his memory, Brandon still had great difficulty in thinking clearly and he experienced problems with balance, which resulted in frequent falls. This was the state Brandon remained in for **35 years** before he saw me.

Since his fetal stem cell treatment, Brandon has kept a written record of his progress. Here are some excerpts. After four months, he reported:

I get stronger and stronger every day and my falling has diminished by 99 percent. I can stand up without the feeling that I'm riding down an elevator.

A short time later Brandon reported:

I can swim for long periods, and I am able to jog now. My vision is 20/20, where before I used to have to wear reading glasses.

My speech has improved, and so has my memory. My reading comprehension is much better, and I've become more aware of the world around me. I've been walking precincts in support of political candidates that I believe will make our country better.

I feel that my confidence is at an all-time high, and as an added benefit, my allergies are all gone.

Six months after Brandon's treatment, his mother wrote:

Here are some of my observations since Brandon came back from his treatment.

Since a month after his treatment, I have seen a continuing maturation in Brandon psychologically. Not only is he now chatting up a storm, but he has also been teasing people, where before he didn't interact much with anyone. He is much more self-directed and self-disciplined, and continues to become a lot more confident as well.

He's much more assertive than he used to be, and continues to develop emotionally, almost as if he is growing up. His progress is occurring by leaps and bounds each month.

Most of all, I enjoy his sense of humor and joy. I didn't realize that I had not heard him laugh for 35 years.

After receiving fetal stem cells, Brandon became active in politics. During the last presidential campaign, he gave several speeches in his community about the stem cell issue, letting people know that he would not have been able to do so were it not for his own stem cell treatment.

Matthew

Matthew was five and a half when his parents first brought him to me. At two weeks of age, Matthew had a devastating reaction to the hepatitis B vaccine. Major areas of his left brain hemisphere and left frontal lobe were damaged, and there was spotty damage to his right hemisphere and frontal lobe. The doctors estimated that in total, roughly 40 percent of his brain was destroyed and there was no hope for recovery.

Within three weeks after receiving the fetal stem cells, his speech therapist noted that Matthew was more attentive and was developing had more interest in learning new words. For the first time, he could say words like "horse," "doggy," and "happy birthday". His physical therapist also noticed that he was much quicker in processing time, and that his attention span had increased.

Three months after Matthew's treatment, his mother wrote:

Matthew continues to master new words and their meanings and his interest in learning has accelerated. Before he received the stem cells, he was so frustrated that he couldn't communicate through words that he just stopped trying. Now he will go to the stereo and say, "I want to dance." Or he will go to the fridge and say, "I want juice." One of the highlights last week was asking him to say, "I love you," and he did it the first time he was asked. My heart just melted!

In a subsequent letter, his mother added:

The biggest difference to report now is how much more quickly Matthew is processing things. He's learning more new words and their meanings every week, repeating them correctly, and making connections with objects in his environment. For example, he loves looking at magazines, and we have been using them as teaching tools for some time now. His vocabulary is really growing, and all of his therapists comment that he is spontaneously talking a lot more and with much better understanding. Physically, he's also doing great.

Six months after his first treatment, Matthew returned for a second. His mother soon wrote:

Since returning home, Matthew has had some of his best days ever. His teachers report that he is happy, talking up a storm and learning better. I am thrilled to see him becoming a more mature little boy.

After another six months, his mother reported:

Matthew continues to make significant progress with his motor skills. Last winter he skied from the top of Vail Mountain on his own. This is a major breakthrough.

Matthew also swam on the swim team three days a week this past summer. He learned to do freestyle and the backstroke, and how to practice in the pool lane with other kids. He also learned how to dive into the pool. It was very exciting!

We have to watch what we say now, or else a little voice might just repeat it. I've heard him say "damn it," or "shoot" when I've forgotten something and had to run back in the house. Just this morning, he was singing parts of Sheryl Crow's song "Soak Up the Sun" while I was driving him to school.

I am so thankful to see him improve both physically and mentally, and so very grateful to you for the fetal stem cells.

Rebecca

In another case, Rebecca, due to anoxia, had been brain damaged since birth. She was brought to me when she was one and a half years old. Her condition necessitated a tracheotomy (a surgical procedures on the neck to open a direct airway through an incision in the trachea (the windpipe.) Past SPECT brain scans revealed that Rebecca's brain activity was far below normal.

Within only three weeks of receiving the cells, Rebecca could breathe without her endotracheal tube, and it was subsequently removed. She also started to show positive changes in both her mental and physical abilities.

Around that time, Rebecca underwent another SPECT brain scan, which, to her doctor's amazement, revealed a 15 percent increase in brain activity. The brain scan confirmed that the fetal stem cells were repairing the damage to her brain. She continues to improve to this day.

Brain Scan Proof

Brain scans of brain-damaged patients—both children and adults— validate the efficacy of fetal stem cell therapy. That is, we observe actual physical changes in the brain in scans.

An example of this is Neil, a 46-year-old attorney who suffered serious brain damage as a result of a mugging. Soon after he received the fetal stem cells, a brain scan engendered the following report from his doctor:

When compared with a brain scan taken prior to the stem cell treatment, it is obvious that significant improvement has taken place, plus, I discern positive changes in his behavior.

All too often, brain-damaged patients are given little or no hope of recovery. But what you have just read are only a few of many examples of the improvements we have seen consistently after fetal stem cell treatment. The improvements these patients have achieved are just the beginning of the progress that lies in their future. I believe that in their lifetimes, especially the children's, there is potential for these patients to become normal.

Cancer

The power to prevent, control and overcome cancer lives within your own immune defense system.

—The Cancer Research Institute

Our bodies are composed of many different types of cells. These cells reproduce themselves to keep up with the demand for function and maintenance of our organs and our general good health. Sometimes, however, this process goes astray, and cells keep dividing even though new cells are not needed. If this process continues, it becomes cancer.

Previously I noted that we develop 250 million cancer and precancerous cells every day, and that our immune systems can usually recognize and destroy these abnormal cells. But as the immune system weakens, either from age or from a physiological insult such as free-radical damage, it becomes progressively less able to control abnormal cell growth. Eventually, these fast-growing cells can form a large mass known as a tumor, or cancer.

Cancer has the unique ability to cloak itself—to hide from the immune system. And as a tumor grows, bits of it can break off and enter the bloodstream or the lymphatic system. These microscopic bits of the original tumor can then migrate to other organs and create new cancers; this process is called metastasis.

Cancer slowly destroys organs, saps the body's energy and resources, and poisons the body with toxic waste products. Left unchecked, the cancer will eventually result in the death of the patient.

In 1971 President Richard Nixon declared a "war on cancer." At that time, it was estimated that one out of every ten Americans was likely to develop cancer in his or her lifetime. Today, according to the National Cancer Institute (NCI), that number has dramatically increased to 50 percent of American men and over 40 percent of American women. It's estimated that more than 1.4 million Americans will be diagnosed with cancer and 560,000 Americans will die of the disease in 2010 alone.

Cancer is the leading cause of death in the United States for people under the age of 85. Survival rates for cancer patients have improved slightly over the last few years, but the "war on cancer" has been a failure, despite the untold billions spent on research.

Once, it was a disease that typically struck individuals in late middle or old age. Today, however, men and women in their 30s and 40s represent one of the fastest-growing age groups apt to develop cancer. And children between the ages of 3 and 13 die from cancer more than from any other disease.

Why are younger people getting cancer at increasing rates? A prevalent theory blames Americans' increasingly toxic diets, obesity reaching alarming record numbers in children, and our environment growing more poisonous every day.

In addition to the obvious human costs, the financial cost for the treatment and care of cancer patients is astronomical.

There is one factor that can contribute significantly to all cancers: a compromised immune system.

For example, even though cancer is the leading cause of death among children 3 to 13, the incidence of cancer among children is far less than for those aged 60 and older. This is the case simply because our immune system is much healthier, stronger, and more effective when we are young; it then declines in effectiveness as we age.

Why Fetal Stem Cell Therapy Is Ideal for Use in Cancer Treatment

The most common method of cancer treatment is chemotherapy. But the side effects can be perilous. Principal among these side effects is a marked weakening of the patients' immune system, rendering them much more vulnerable to infections and other diseases. Consequently, some reputable studies have concluded that more people die from their chemo-therapy treatment than from their original cancer.

Donor bone marrow stem cell transplants are used to treat certain types of cancers, such as leukemia. These transplants require the use of immunosuppressives, drugs that suppress the patient's immune system to prevent the donor cells from attacking the recipient. Once again, this is known as the potentially fatal, graft-versus-host disease.

It is reported that even when there is a perfect donor match and the perfect amount of immunosuppressive drugs are administered, 25 percent of these patients will still die.

In what are called autologous stem cell transplants, the stem cells are taken from the patients themselves, then "cleaned" and returned to the patient. In this method of treatment, however, some of the cancer cells escape the "cleaning" and are present among the cells returned to the patient. These returned cancer cells are more virulent, more therapy-resistant than typical cancer cells, because they were powerful enough to survive the cleaning process. When these resistant cells are returned to the patient's body, a cancer of an even more aggressive type can develop; I call this "Secondary Cancer."

You have already read how all the problems I have just discussed can be completely avoided through the use of fetal stem cells.

Fetal stem cells do not have antigenicity, which means that no one must die for lack of a donor match, because of a suppressed immune system, or because cancerous cells are transferred back into the patient. And as previously noted, fetal stem cells actually constitute a new immune system that's at least 10 times more powerful than the native immune system of a normal, healthy adult.

Fetal stem cells not only function as replacements for impaired immune cells; they also *stimulate the body's own cells* to multiply and attack the cancer.

Fetal stem cells are unique in another crucial way. They possess an *internal system of quality-control screening* that prevents any abnormalities and malformations from being passed from them to the recipient.

In summary, here are the ways in which fetal stem cells are beneficial in the treatment of cancer:

- Bolster the patient's *own original* immune system so that it is stronger than it was before the patient became ill, rather than being compromised by the illness.
- Provide a new *immune system* that is at least 10 times stronger than that of a normal, healthy one.
- Significantly reduce or even *eliminate the side-effects* of traditional cancer treatments.
- *Hasten recovery time.*

- *Eliminate the problems of bone marrow transplants*—including weakened immune system, graft-versus-host disease, and donor matching.

- Can be *administered as many times as is necessary* to help ensure a recovery from cancer, because they have no cellular fingerprint, and the supply of fetal stem cells is virtually unlimited.

- Allow stronger doses of chemotherapy to be used, with no negative side effect.

Using Every Weapon to Fight Cancer

When I began treating patients with fetal stem cells, one of my cancer patients told me that she refused to undergo any conventional cancer treatments. She insisted on fetal stem cell treatment only. I tried to convince her that she should avail herself of all traditional and alternative methods available, but she was unyielding. Her diagnosis was early-stage breast cancer.

After receiving the fetal stem cells, she went into remission and has remained cancer-free ever since.

Does this mean I recommend fetal stem cell therapy as an alternative to other cancer treatments? Absolutely not. This woman was very lucky, in my opinion, because by insisting that fetal stem cells be her only form of treatment, she limited her chances for recovery.

Today I will not allow my cancer patients to receive fetal stem cell treatment unless they also obtain other synergistic, ancillary treatments appropriate for their specific disease.

The following are some of what I consider to be synergistic, with the fetal cells, in the treatment of cancer. Unfortunately, most of them are not available in the United States:

- *Hyperthermia*

  Hyperthermia involves the localized or systemic application of heat.

  Tumors, due to their rapid abnormal growth, require ever-increasing nourishment, which is supplied by the growth of many new arteries to supply blood (nourishment) to the tumor. However, the veins that carry blood away from the tumor remain normal in size and number.

  If you heat a given area, the normal tissue takes in the heat through its arteries and then releases it through its veins. But in a tumor, with its expanded inflow of blood, heat arrives at an accelerated rate—building up faster than it can be expelled through the tumor's "normal" venous system. In a sense, the tumor then becomes a heat sink.

  Not only does this mechanism provide for the destruction of the cancer, but if any tumor should remain it has now become vulnerable to a smaller and much less toxic dose of chemotherapy.

  Although hyperthermia is safe, effective and has been successfully used in other countries such as Germany for over 35 years, there are very few treatment facilities using hyperthermia in the United States. Why? In my opinion it is because hyperthermia is nowhere at all as profitable, as compared to conventional cancer treatments such as chemotherapy.

- *Boosting natural killer cells*

Another cancer-fighting tactic that is synergistic with fetal stem cells is to boost the number of natural killer (NK) cells, which are the cells of our immune-system that directly attack cancer.

- *Chemosensitivity tests*

Another option in the treatment of cancer that should be used more frequently by oncologists is chemosensitivity testing.

Standard chemotherapy is a kind of "cookbook" procedure. You have diagnosis X—the medical textbook says to administer chemotherapy B. Chemosensitivity testing fine-tunes the chemotherapy to the ideal drug choice and dosage for maximum effectiveness in destroying the cancer in that individual patient.

To accomplish this, the doctor extracts the patient's own unique cancer cells from the bloodstream and then grows them in a laboratory. Once the cells are grown, the oncologist adds various chemotherapies and combinations thereof to find *the treatment that is most effective in destroying that unique cancer.*

- *Cancer markers*

Another weapon in the anticancer arsenal is the use of cancer markers. Before a tumor has grown to the point that it is discernible on scans, such as an MRI, a simple blood test for tumor-specific markers indicates whether or not the cancer is being destroyed, which is a very early sign of if the chosen chemotherapy combination is working or, if not, should be changed.

- *Benign agents*

Many simple and benign agents—mistletoe, aged garlic extract, glutathiomine and snail extract among others—are successful in the treatment of cancer without any harmful side effects. Again, such therapies are used mostly outside the United States.

All of the above-mentioned cancer treatment options are synergistic with the use of fetal stem therapy, as are many others.

With that said, let me present a few case histories of my cancer patients.

Joanne

Joanne represents a perfect example of the unique power of fetal stem cells to significantly reduce the side effects of chemotherapy. When Joanne told her oncologist she was going to receive fetal stem cells before starting her high-dose chemotherapy regime, he told her that she was being foolish and wasting her money.

After receiving her first high-dose chemotherapy treatment, instead of experiencing the predicted negative side effects her oncologist had warned her about, she felt fine. In fact, she told him, she was very hungry and anxious to leave the hospital to go to her favorite restaurant. Her doctor told her that the lack of side effects was unusual and she was very lucky. He added that the next round of chemotherapy would probably "hit her like a ton of bricks."

But the second round of chemotherapy also produced no significant negative side effects. Joanne completed the full course of chemotherapy sessions and went into remission without experiencing any of the major negative side effects which are common during such an intense course of treatment.

Ralph

Ralph had been diagnosed with an advanced stage of resistant Hodgkin's disease.

Treated at a highly respected cancer clinic, Ralph showed no improvement after his chemotherapy and began to deteriorate rapidly. His prognosis was grim. He was told that nothing more could be done for him and that he had only a matter of a few more weeks to live.

Because the hospital was outside the United States, I was able to offer both Ralph and his oncologist his only possible option—an "experimental" treatment plan using fetal stem cells. We would give Ralph the fetal stem cells and then administer myelotoxic chemotherapy, a level of chemotherapy considered to be a potentially lethal overdose by conventional medical standards.

The doctors warned Ralph that he likely would not survive the assault on his immune system, but because it was his only hope, Ralph chose to moved forward with the procedure.

After his first fetal stem cell treatment, Ralph was given his first dose—or overdose—of chemotherapy. Incredibly, his blood counts bounced back to normal levels within five days. Ralph received two more courses of fetal stem cells before the next two doses of myelotoxic chemotherapy. Again, within five days, all his blood counts returned to normal levels.

Ralph's oncologists checked the status of his resistant Hodgkin's disease using a full battery of tests and determined that he was in complete remission—*a result never before reported in the medical literature*. Four days after his last chemotherapy, Ralph was discharged from the hospital.

In their medical report, Ralph's oncologists wrote: "The fetal stem cell transplantation has allowed us to treat a terminal resistant Hodgkin's disease patient, with an extremely myelotoxic chemotherapy regimen successfully, while eliminating its potentially fatal complications."

Ralph was treated over six years ago. He regularly receives quarterly check-ups, including lab studies, to monitor his progress. His cancer remains in *complete remission*.

Alice

Alice was diagnosed with stage 3 ovarian cancer and received high-dose chemotherapy. One month after receiving fetal stem cells, Alice wrote:

I had my first blood test last Monday. It's been only one month since I got the fetal stem cells and for the first time since I don't remember when, I have normal white and red cell counts. That got the attention of the medical group, who found it impossible to believe.

Even better than that is how I feel: I have soooooo much energy right now that it is baffling. And I am hungry all the time. I eat probably seven small meals every day.

My skin has completely changed. All the dark chemo spots are going away. My complexion is reverting back to younger days. All my wrinkles are going away. My skin is so smooth.

Also my libido has gone through the roof. My boyfriend has been quoted as saying that he may have to get a backup plan as he may not be able to handle me. And for him to say that is something!

Everyone that sees me is amazed at the rapid changes. I actually had someone ask me what kind of illicit drugs I was taking, as I have so much energy. I don't remember feeling this good ever.

I cannot thank you enough.

Janet

Janet was only two years old when her parents brought her to me. She had been diagnosed with brain cancer.

After chemotherapy produced no improvement, the oncologist informed Janet's parents that he could do no more because, due to its location, her tumor was inoperable

After exhausting all medical alternatives, her parents decided to try fetal stem cell treatment.

Six weeks after Janet received the cells, her mother wrote:

Janet is really doing great and we're happy with what we've seen so far and are very hopeful for what is to come. The first improvement we noticed was with Janet's vision. Typically she would roll her eyes up in her head. She doesn't do this anymore. I can call her name and she looks right at me. And she can hold her stare. She tracks back and forth and really watches what's going on around her. She's smiling much more often, too, and is much happier. She's even gotten so excited at times that she's giggled, which she never did before.

By William C. Rader, MD

Janet is now beginning to vocalize for the first time and is trying very hard to talk. She responds with sounds when we talk with her, obviously now comprehending what we are saying and communicating back to us. She's getting real close to saying "Mama," which means so much to me.

Her motor skills are improving as well. She is now really moving around a lot and is able to kick her feet and move her arms much better. When we place her on her knees, she holds them up under her, whereas before they would just slide out from underneath her. She is also now able to extend her arms forward to reach for things like her toys. She can even turn her battery-powered toys on and off on command!

Her appetite is noticeably increased, she's eating extremely well, and is starting to gain weight. She's sleeping well, too, much better than before she received the fetal stem cells.

Janet's improvements continued over the next two years, during which time she received one additional fetal stem cell treatment.

In a recent letter, Janet's mother reported: "It's now over two years since Janet's initial stem cell treatment. In all this time, she has continually improved to the point where her brain tumor hasn't had any negative effect whatsoever."

While I cannot say for certain that the fetal stem cells destroyed Janet's tumor, I can say with certainty that after she received the cells, the symptoms of her brain tumor began to turn around—and now her physicians consider the tumor to be inactive. In fact, her mother's told me the oncologist's exact words were that it had become a "dead" tumor.

Beth

Beth was diagnosed with breast cancer, and after undergoing an extensive regimen of chemotherapy followed by radiation therapy, she chose fetal stem cell therapy. What follows is the progress report she sent to me.

I received the fetal stem cells twice. The first time was four weeks after completing seven months of chemotherapy and radiation for my breast cancer. I believe the cells helped speed along my recovery and the return of my high level of energy, so much so that I have been able to return to my favorite sport, skiing.

The second time I received the stem cells was 18 months later. Since then, I can honestly say that I feel as good now as I did when I was 30, and I'm about to turn 55!

Besides dealing with my cancer, another example of how the stem cells are doing their job is related to a severe tibia-fibula spiral fracture of my left leg that occurred while I was skiing, which required having a titanium rod installed in my tibia. My surgeon said it would take a full year or more for a complete healing, provided that the bone healed at all. My healing process was outstanding, and because I healed so quickly my surgeon released me from his care in six months!

I returned to skiing and my first run was black diamond, the most difficult run! I attribute this directly to the fetal stem cells, as I do, more importantly, the fact that my blood work continues to improve each time that I see my oncologist. I've been cancer-free for three years now.

Hurray!

By William C. Rader, MD

Here are some excerpts from reports sent by other patients of mine who made fetal stem cell therapy an integral part of their cancer treatment:

Carol, breast cancer:

I was diagnosed with stage 4 breast cancer. I had five tumors, each about four centimeters, in my lymph nodes. Through chemotherapy, all five tumors were reduced in size, but they did not go away. I lived with that condition for two years. Then I received the fetal stem cells. Four months later, I had my follow up CT scan. All the lesions were gone.

Allen, prostate cancer:

"After receiving the stem cells, my latest prostate biopsy was negative. My oncologist is still scratching his head. He doesn't understand why my prostate is now free of the cancer."

John, pancreatic cancer:

"It's been almost two and half years since I was first diagnosed with pancreatic cancer. Because of the combination of the superb treatment I received from my oncologist and the fetal stem cells, I am a survivor."

Betty, thyroid cancer:

"Since receiving the stem cells, my chest feels more open, allowing me to breathe more easily. I have fewer incidences of choking and problems swallowing. My voice is stronger too. Although he felt it to

be very unusual, my physician thinks that my laryngeal nerve has reconnected. The remaining lobe of my thyroid is producing at normal levels and my energy levels are much higher."

Mac, leiomyosarcoma (cancer of the smooth muscle):

"My oncologist was amazed at the positive changes in the CRP (C-reactive protein, a cancer marker) within only a few weeks after receiving the fetal stem cells."

Dorothy, breast cancer:

"After my chemotherapy my hemoglobin level dropped to 6.4. I was given three pints of blood, and I received an injection of Procrit once a week to help increase my red blood cell count. After receiving the fetal stem cells, all my blood counts returned to normal. It's been more than five years since my first stem cell treatment. (Dorothy was treated twice). My cancer has not returned and my blood counts have remained stable."

An Experiment

In an attempt to prove the inherent ability of fetal stem cells to seek out and destroy cancer cells, we performed an experiment in my laboratory. A Petri dish containing nutrients was prepared. Four circular holes were punched into the plate to form four round wells. As shown in Figure 1, one hole was punched in the center of the plate and the remaining three were punched around the circumference of the plate at 9, 12, and 3 o'clock, respectively.

- The 9 o'clock well was filled with normal cells.
- The 12 o'clock well was filled with an average form of cancer cells.
- The 3 o'clock well was filled with an extremely severe form of cancer cells.

Fetal stem cells were labeled with a fluorescent dye that emits visible light when placed under ultraviolet light, and then placed in the center well. The dish was placed under ultraviolet light for observation.

The fetal stem cells migrated from the center well to various areas of the Petri dish, as seen in Figure 2:

1. Essentially *none* of the fetal stem cells migrated toward the normal cells.
2. Approximately *30 percent* of the fetal stem cells migrated to the average cancer cells.
3. Approximately *70 percent* of the fetal stem cells migrated to the extremely severe cancer cells.

Over time, the fetal stem cells then destroyed all the cancer cells.

Cancer

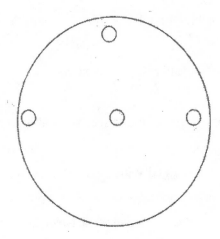

Figure 1

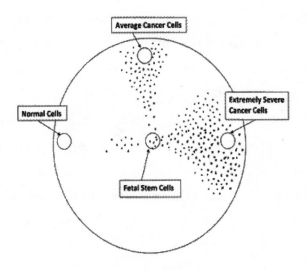

Figure 2

Once again, I cannot say with certainty that the fetal stem cell treatment is responsible for all the improvements and remissions you have just read about. As said earlier, I insist that all of my cancer patients pursue conventional or alternative treatments, or both, in addition to receiving fetal stem cells.

Nevertheless, I consistently see irrefutably positive results that far exceed the statistical rates of success for patients with similar cancers.

Because it can markedly increase immune system function, fetal stem cell therapy has an enormous potential for preventing cancer within all of us. Fetal stem cells are therefore a two-edged sword in the fight against cancer: They reduce the chances of getting cancer, and they effect significant measurable improvements in the treatment outcomes of those who have cancer.

Fetal stem cells possess superior strength compared to any other stem cell, enabling them to ward off the toxicity of chemotherapy. Also a patient can receive them an unlimited number of times during and after chemotherapy. These inherent qualities of the fetal stem cell allow a cancer patient to receive essentially unrestricted amounts of chemotherapy, which can then eventually destroy the tumor.

Could fetal stem cells then be the "super weapon" against all cancers that we have been searching for these many years?

Cerebral Palsy

Cerebral palsy affects about 400,000 children and adults in the United States. It is caused by damage to one or more specific areas of the brain. The most common cause is deprivation of oxygen in the brain of a fetus or newborn baby. *cause*

    Common symptoms include speech impairment, muscle tightness or spasm, involuntary movements, severe disturbances in gait and mobility, and in some cases delayed cognitive development and seizures. Today, conventional and alternative medicines offer cerebral palsy patients nothing more than minimal relief from their symptoms.

    Although cerebral palsy is considered to be a lifelong, incurable disease, patients treated with fetal stem cell therapy have had dramatic positive outcomes, as evidenced by the following progress reports I have received from the parents of my cerebral palsy patients.

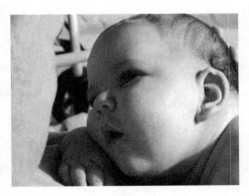

Chris

    When Chris was brought to me for treatment for his Cerebral Palsy, he was only 10 months old. At birth, he suffered from lack of oxygen for an extended period, resulting in multiple strokes and severe brain damage. The following is Chris's history as written by his mother:

Chris was born December 18th, 2008 at 8:42am via repeat c-section. His cry was the most beautiful sound ever and then he was sent back to our room. On his way to our room he started grunting.

After checking him, the nurse immediately rushed him to the Neonatal ICU (NICU). When they let me see him, he was already on a ventilator. What a scary thought for any mom. Little did I know that was just the beginning.

I was told to go back to my room and try to get some sleep. I had no idea why I was having such trouble sleeping until a nurse came barging through my door saying the NICU needs to talk to you ASAP. I immediately called the NICU nurse. She said, "I just wanted you to know that he is not doing so well on his ventilator and we are going to have to switch him over to a higher powered ventilator, you don't need to come down here I just wanted to let you know what we were doing." Needless to say I had the nurse help me get down there right away.

When I got to the NICU there were 3 nurses working with Chris and you could just look at his face and tell he was not doing well. A doctor that I had never met came over to me and said, "Chris would likely need to be transferred to another hospital for a procedure called ECMO, which is a heart lung machine for newborns." He immediately ordered for med-flight to transfer Chris.

He arrived at the new hospital at 7:30am. He was 47 hours old. We were immediately greeted by the Pediatric Surgeons who informed us that Chris had "coded" on the elevator, but they were able to get his heart restarted.

We were told that his only chance at survival was to be immediately put on the ECMO machine.

Four hours later a nurse came out and simply said, "It is not good. He had coded 2 more times and suffered a large liver laceration from the CPR chest compressions and as a result he had a massive blood loss and to prepare ourselves." This was the first and last time I said to myself, "Are we doing the right thing? Should we stop fighting? Does he want us to let him go?" The priest was called to our room and I couldn't even speak to him. I was so angry with god.

About 1 hour later the Pediatric Surgeon came into our room and as soon as she saw us she wept. She explained that Chris would be a minute-by-minute little boy. That while they were putting the tubes into his Carotid and Jugular veins to hook up the ECMO machine, that he coded again and because of the blood pressure drop his Carotid and Jugular veins were shredded. (I couldn't believe she used the word shredded). She went on to explain "because of that they had to open his chest and put the tubes directly through his heart."

She then explained to us that we would have to prepare ourselves that his chest was open with tubes sticking out and that his abdomen was left open and that if he survived he would need several more surgeries to repair the liver laceration.

There is NO!!!! preparation for this.

When we arrived in the ICU he was swollen and purple. The metallic smell was horrifying. He was bleeding extensively. He was lying in so much blood, that the nurses had to change his bedding every 15-30

By William C. Rader, MD

minutes. He was lifeless. Our surgeon asked if we minded if she go to the chapel and pray for him.

We stayed by his bedside over night. The next morning we were just breathing a sigh of relief that he had made it through the night. The nurse said that his ultrasound results of his head were back and they were not good and that the doctors wanted to meet with us at 10:30 am.

At the meeting, we were told that we had two choices; either let him go, or try to put him back on the ventilator.

They said if he survived he would absolutely have CP and many developmental problems.

I looked at my son and said, "Chris mommy and daddy love you and we understand if you are tired and want to go home, but if you are willing to fight I do not care how many people in this room don't believe in you, Mom and Dad will fight as hard as we can."

Well evidentially he wanted to fight because even on all of his sedatives and pain meds, he opened his eyes real big and starred into my eyes for what seemed like an eternity.

The hospital called in the priest (my husband could not handle this. He screamed across the room when he saw him, "Get Out!!!") They also called the "post mortem photographer". She was to take pictures of Chris if he did not make it.

Needless to say he did not die. He lived. The photographer asked if we still wanted her to take pictures. I said absolutely not. In my mind it was bad karma. She was there to take a certain picture and if I gave in, perhaps Chris would also.

At that point, the surgeons came back into the room. To add insult to injury they never thought he would survive, so they did not think about what to do if he did make it.

Chris never looked back. He was off of all supplemental oxygen within the next 3 weeks. He had 6 more surgeries in the next week. Meaning in his first 10 days of life, he had endured 7 surgeries.

An MRI of his brain showed "Near complete replacement of bilateral cerebral hemispheres due to liquefaction necrosis from global ischemia". Words I will never forget. It meant: most of his brain had been destroyed. The doctors strongly cautioned us not to take Chris home, saying that "He would be our sleeping baby until he died." And they even had the nerve to ask us if we realized what this could do to our other two children, if we were to take him home.

We took Chris home and started our journey

Chris made no noise at all. He was only awake about 5-10 minutes every 6-8 hours. We were noticing more and more spasticity every day. He was fighting so hard but his little body was starting to give in to his brain damage

Every time I took Chris to the doctor I was questioned as to why we chose to take him home. I even said to my husband, "It feels like with each appointment I am punched in the gut."

Chris was being treated by his doctor for his seizure disorder. One day at the doctor's office we were saying how we know that we need to treat his seizures but we wanted to make sure that we did not over treat and sedate him, because we knew that if we were going to get any neurological function back, over sedating him would interfere with any possible recovery. She actually chuckled and said "You do not need to worry about sedating him; it is not as if he is going to learn anything anyway." We immediately changed Neurologists.

We received the results of Chris's next brain scan. It was horrible. Chris's strokes had spread and it destroyed more than 65% of his brain. Funny...my question to the Neurologist was, "Ok so now that the damage is done there is nothing that we can do, no surgery, nothing? Just watch him die?"

Ironically, the Neurologist said "Well, barring going to China."

She assured me that "IF" it were proven to be a successful treatment, in just a matter of time it would be available in the United States and that we should just wait.

I was NOT ok with waiting, so I started researching on my own, calling Wake Forrest University, Duke, Harvard, Stanford, St Jude Children's Hospital and MD Anderson. Only MD Anderson would even talk to me. The doctor there said even if the U.S. were eventually going to do anything, they wouldn't touch a patient like Chris.

Little did he know that what he said energized me even more. I kept researching and found MEDRA. The more I read the more excited I became. I spoke with your offices and the employees who themselves were parents of a brain damaged child. I knew this was our only chance.

Bob and I finally decided that worst case scenario...I would rather take a chance and nothing was to happen, than not take a chance and lose him.

Thanks to your generosity Chris got his first set of cells on June 27th, 2009 (his daddy's birthday). What a birthday present!!!

We did not see much the first 4 weeks. Then came 6 weeks post stem cells... Every day we were getting progressions. Chris started making noises (he was totally non-verbal before) he would fuss, his suck reflexes were stronger, his muscles were less rigid, we could actually open his hands and he could lay them flat, his was lifting his head from the floor using his arms. With each day came more and more.

He eventually started sitting up by himself, rolling over, trying to stand up and when put on his tummy, he would start moving his legs one right after the other and lifting his upper body trying to crawl. I could not believe this was the same baby.

Chris was initially diagnosed with Cortical Blindness, his pupils had been pin point and totally non-reactive ever since the strokes. About 2 ½ months after our first set of cells we were sitting at home and out of the blue his pupils were dilated and he became agitated. At first I was scared that it might be another stroke; however when I pointed a flashlight at him, his pupils reacted. I couldn't believe it. He kept this up for about 3 hours, before he ended up falling asleep. His pupils have continued to do this since.

Dr. Rader when you first spoke to us after looking at Chris's medical records, you said that Chris would be best served with 3-4 treatments spaced out every 3-6 months because of the degree of his brain damage. We returned for his 2nd set of cells only 4 months later. Pretty incredible that we saw that much progress in only 4 months ... hah?

When we got to the hotel we called you because of how bad his seizures had gotten during the trip. It was amazing; you sent a doctor, a nurse and a medical assistant to our room, to take care of Chris within minutes. They all stayed, continually checking in with you, for more than 2 hours until Chris's seizures calmed down.

Within days of that second treatment, Chris's seizures had gone from 50 plus per day to 10 to 20. Within only 4 weeks we went from 10 to 20 per day to on most days none and on a bad day a maximum of 5. We started weaning him off of one of his 3 seizure medicines on day 27 post cells. It took us about 3 weeks to get him completely off of his medications. However he handled it flawlessly, with NO increase in seizures. He is now having days with no seizures at all.

His suck and swallow are getting better. He is even taking a pacifier. Chris is getting so vocal that he has even woke us up at night on a couple occasions. He is fighting off his own infections and illnesses.

For the first time in his life, he is now able to see!!! He even strained his head back to see the Christmas tree that was behind him. His vision therapist when asked what to get him for Christmas said, "Anything that he can see, he is definitely not blind." Last week he reached out his hand to touch a green balloon. This was his first time ever he reached out to touch something.

Also Chris has had a hearing aide that he has worn since he was 4 months old for a hearing loss in his left ear. Today his hearing was tested and it was normal. No more hearing aide. Yaay! I hope this news makes you smile half as much as it does us.

Chris met our biggest goal on December 18th, 2009...He had his first birthday! Back when Chris was 4 months old and we got his CT scan, we were told his life expectancy was only 9 months to 1 year max. One of his nurses came to his 1st birthday party. She sat there for almost 2 hours holding him. When I sat down with her she said, "I am just in awe over him...He just shouldn't be here, he is truly a miracle." She went on to say that "Chris is the talk of her shift. She of course is not allowed to recommend stem cells. However she has been telling parents of her patients to remain determined to make the best of their child's life no matter what the doctors say."

We are so excited to see what he will do in the weeks to come.

I have been exposed to the most amazing people through this incredible time in our life.

Needless to say...YOU HAVE GIVEN US OUR BABY BACK!!! But most of all YOU HAVE GIVEN MIKE AND JACK THEIR BROTHER BACK!!!

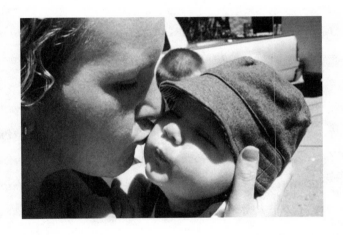

Thanks to you and your company we were able to have a Christmas with our baby. Also thanks to you, we were able to look in the face of one of the doctors who offered no help and only limitations, a doctor who said Chris would never make it to 1 year and hold our tongues, while we giggled at his 1 year WELL CHILD check up.

Marisa

Marisa was four and a half years old when we first met. She had suffered with cerebral palsy all her life. Because of her severe lack of coordination and her muscle spasms, Marisa needed a child's walker just to achieve very limited mobility. She was prone to falling forward, and was in constant fear of doing so, even when sitting. Also, Marisa's speech was so difficult to understand that she would become extremely frustrated when she attempted to communicate.

Three months after Marisa received fetal stem cells, her mother sent me this progress report:

I'm excited to report that we've seen a dramatic increase in Marisa's speech and mobility. We can now understand her words 100 percent better than before. Her ability to ambulate in her walker has increased as well. When Marisa is standing in her walker or sitting independently, she is much more relaxed and is more steady, secure, and comfortable with her actions. Prior to receiving the fetal stem cells, she had a constant fear of falling. Now, if she is sitting and loses her balance, she is able to catch herself and, if need be, put herself back up to a sitting position.

Marisa is now able to move across the floor on her buttocks and is also learning how to crawl. Her hand and arm movements have increased phenomenally. For the first time, she is able to write her name! She has also made dramatic improvements in her ability to feed herself.

There are so many other improvements that our family, friends, and teachers have noticed in Marisa since she received the fetal stem cells that they are too numerous to mention.

We are eagerly anticipating what new surprises lay ahead for Marisa and our family.

Eric

Eric was diagnosed with cerebral palsy when he was six months old. He was extremely spastic, drooled constantly, and could not move about on his own.

Eric's cognitive abilities were also significantly affected. He had great difficulty making sense of what he was told, and he was unable to express himself.

Eric first received fetal stem cell therapy when he was three years old. Afterward, his mother wrote:

The day after Eric received the fetal stem cells he started crawling on all fours. This is something he had never been able to do before, though he'd tried many times. And since then, he's just gotten better and better.

Another important change we noticed soon after his treatment was that Eric's cognitive ability dramatically improved. He is now following commands and is also for the first time making some commands of his own. He's expressing his likes and dislikes, and it's obvious that he knows what's going on around him. Wherever the other kids are is where he has to be now, something that was never the case before his treatment.

The other day, the other children all went outside to play, and I picked him up, because he was heading out the door yelling, "Outside, outside!" over and over. I love it.

In her next progress report, Eric's mother wrote:

Overall, Eric is communicating so much better. He is now capable of giving us high fives! Last week he also started to wave. He's trying to teach himself how to use a spoon to eat. He can already get the spoon to his mouth, though he can't dip it into food yet. But he's trying hard, and before he couldn't even manage to hold the spoon. Now he is able to maneuver his toys and no longer drools at all! Eric has become a very happy, content child who loves to play. Since his treatment, he enjoys calling out to each family member by name while balancing himself standing on the couch.

Eric is also exhibiting many positive changes at school—so many that they have decided to videotape him so they can keep track of them all. Both his teacher and I have noticed how much better he is at paying attention. In the past he didn't look at you when you spoke to him. Today in class he would turn his head and look at each child when they spoke. His teacher said he was really soaking it all in.

He's very excited and enthusiastic about his progress, and really making a strong effort to say new words.

I am so proud of him! He's such a precious child and shows so much determination.

Ben

When his parents first brought him to me, Ben was 12 years old and had suffered from cerebral palsy all his life. His arms were severely contracted, and he could not open his hands. In addition to the common symptoms of cerebral palsy, he suffered from seizures characterized by violent backward head thrusts. His vision was poor, and he seemed oblivious to his surroundings. He didn't speak and rarely looked at people when they spoke to him. His height and weight were far below normal for his age.

After Ben received fetal stem cells, his mother reported:

There's been a marked reduction in Ben's overall spasticity and limb contraction. His hands are now opened and relaxed, and his arms are loose. He is now able to lift his cup and spoon and bring them to his mouth.

His backward head thrusts, which were significant, are also now almost totally gone, and his vision has improved enormously.

The first thing that people who haven't seen Ben for awhile notice is that he immediately turns his head when someone walks into the room. He's also much better able to hold his head up and is eating more solid foods.

Since his treatment, Ben has gained four pounds. He had not gained any weight at all in the entire year before the stem cells. He's also grown three inches in height. Ben is a much happier child, a different child, who continues to communicate and is far less frustrated and more vocal.

For the first time ever, the other day he looked at me and said, "Mama."! I can't begin to tell you what that meant to me.

Marylou

By William C. Rader, MD

Marylou suffered from cerebral palsy from the time she was born. Prior to receiving fetal stem cells at age 10, Marylou never made direct eye contact, rarely spoke, had difficulty comprehending and following simple instructions, tired easily, and had very poor balance. She would back into a chair, feeling her way, in order to seat herself safely.

After Marylou's treatment, her mother reported:

Marylou's reaction within hours was significant. She now makes eye-to-eye contact and looks at things with intention and purpose. On the way home from the clinic, as we awaited our flight at the airport, Marylou pulled away from me and walked 20 feet. Then she looked at a chair, and instead of backing into it, she sat down normally. This was a definite first.

Once home, Marylou went into the bathroom and closed the door behind her, something else she has never done before.

Since then, she continues to make noticeable improvements in her overall behavior. She is beginning to vocalize more and more and now is able to use speech in proper context. In the past, instead of true conversations, she would imitate whoever spoke to her and always spoke of herself in the third person, beginning her sentences with "Marylou," instead of "I." Now, without prompting, she is initiating conversations and saying "I," instead of her name.

In the next follow up letter, Marylou's mother wrote:

Her balance and endurance have both particularly improved, and more positive changes in these areas are constantly occurring. She now walks/runs three miles, and she is able to follow instructions. She performs simple tasks and does as she is told. For example, I can tell her to turn the light on or off, close the door, go to her room, go outside, take her plate to the sink, and so forth, and she is able to easily comply.

Last week, Marylou underwent an EEG (an electroencephalogram, a test measuring brain wave activity). This is the first time in her life that she has had any normal output in her EEG.

Jimmy

Jimmy's cerebral palsy was a result of his premature birth. At the age of three and a half, his eyesight, comprehension, and ability to speak and eat were greatly affected. Following his first fetal stem cell treatment, his parents wrote:

Jimmy's eyesight continues to improve greatly and the doctor is very impressed with the progress he is making.

Jimmy has also been improving in his ability to eat solid food. His appetite is better and he is now willing to try anything we are eating.

His comprehension continues to get better as well, and he's become so much more vocal. He is now able to say hi, bye, mom, dad, papa, and other words that previously he either did not know or could not pronounce. He is getting stronger every day.

Both of us, as well as his therapists, are very excited by his rapid and continued progress.

By William C. Rader, MD

Bruce and Johnny

Bruce and Johnny are identical twins who were both born with cerebral palsy. They were five years old when I met them.

Three weeks after their treatment, they were evaluated by their pediatrician. The following excerpt is from his report:

Immediate changes in muscle tone in both boys, as well as increased control of facial and mandible (jaw) muscles, opening of their hands, which were previously contracted, better use of upper and lower extremities, a decrease in spasticity of the hips, and better control of the trunk. ... I feel these changes will allow for a cascade of functional improvements.

In a later follow-up progress report, their mother wrote:

Both of the twins continue to make steady improvement, and they are continually doing new things. Among their significant improvements since they received the fetal stem cells are their attention span and motor skills, which are now fine. They can now look at and identify objects by sight, which they could not do before, and they know how to put their fingers out to touch and grasp a switch to enable a device.

Overall, their mental abilities have improved. Now they are able to process what they hear or see or feel. Both boys have come so far that they were well enough to attend our public school's special education classes this term.

Bruce and Johnny have also undergone physical changes. Both of them have improved their sitting balance ability, using their hands for support. Before, they could not sit up by themselves at all. Instead, they would fall over.

Another important benefit from the fetal stem cells is their ability to remain in their leg braces for five hours a day without pain. The braces help them stretch their Achilles tendons and calf muscles and flex their feet. Without the braces, their feet extend straight out, as if they are a continuation of their legs. Before, it was so painful for them that they could only wear the braces for a short period of time. Now, for them to be able to wear them for several hours is a huge improvement, and it is helping their legs and feet return to normal.

The boys are less frustrated because of the improvements in their abilities to communicate. They are able to express themselves better and make themselves understood. Johnny, who was diagnosed as partially blind, now has improvements in his vision.

Both of my boys have reached a level of achievement that far exceeds their original hopeless prognosis, and it's all thanks to the stem cells.

Arthur

Dear Dr. Rader,

The following is a summary of my son Arthur's medical history.

Arthur was born prematurely at 29 weeks of gestation. Shortly thereafter he was diagnosed with cerebral palsy.

As he was growing up he suffered from many of the symptoms of C.P.

He was non verbal.

He had very limited fine motor skills resulting in the inability to pick up objects such as a spoon to feed himself.

His muscles were tight and spastic causing contractions in his shoulders, arms, wrists and his left arm was usually contorted backwards.

He was unable to hold up his head or have control of his upper body. Thus he was unable to sit independently or use any type of adaptive walker.

He became easily fatigued from any type of exertion.

His growth was very slow. His pediatrician put him at less than 25% of normal growth and he also was significantly underweight.

He was extremely sensitive to sounds which made it very difficult for him to sleep.

He would gag almost constantly. When he tried to eat, due to gagging, he suffered from continuous vomiting. The doctors were insisting that I would give them permission to have a feeding tube permanently surgically implanted in Arthur's stomach. I refused to subject him to that and began feeding him myself. I cannot begin to tell you how devastating it was for me to watch my precious son struggle to swallow just a teaspoon of food and then stand by helplessly as he would vomit. But I refused to give in which then would not have allowed him to develop the ability to eat by mouth.

Due to his physical disabilities and the fact that his cognitive skills were so low, he had to be placed in a special school.

Cerebral Palsy

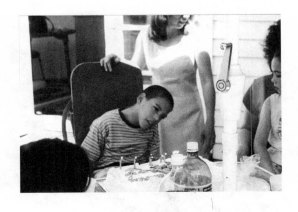

This was Arthur's condition when I brought him to see you 8 years ago.

Since being treated with the fetal stem cells I now have a completely different son.

His growth rate has increased to the 100th percentile. He is very healthy, strong and his body looks like a football player.

He never gags anymore. His favorite food is grilled steak, french fries, crusty french bread and all you can eat salad bars.

Although he still has some difficulties in his speech and fine motor skills his stamina is strong and he no longer becomes fatigued, he actually works 13 hour-days every day and sleeps like a baby for 7 to 8 hours a night.

What is most exciting is the improvements in his cognitive abilities.

*Arthur was transferred to a regular school and graduated from high school as an **honor student**. Additionally, he earned a 5 (highest score) on the AP Calculus exam and now is a freshman at State University where he is currently on the **Dean's list for earning straight A's**.*

I am so proud of him!

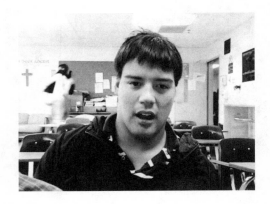

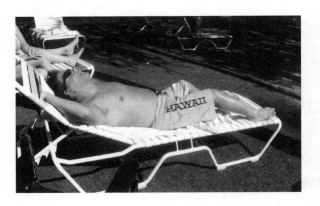

Many thanks for your dedication to these children; your efforts will always be remembered.

Nathan

Nathan was born with a severe form of cerebral palsy that left him completely deaf and unable to speak. His illness appeared so serious and intractable that when Nathan was 10 years old his doctor told his mother that she was wasting her time trying to help him. The doctor said there was no hope for Nathan and recommended that she institutionalize him.

Nathan's mother refused to heed this advice and for years kept looking for a solution. After trying many treatments without success, she learned of the work I was doing.

Four months after receiving fetal stem cells, Nathan was able to hear and speak for the first time.

Mindy

Mindy also was severely affected by cerebral palsy. When I first met her, her eyes were rolled back to the point where only a small portion of her irises were visible. No matter who spoke to her, even her parents, her eyes remained frozen in this position.

After Mindy received the fetal stem cells, her mother reported:

Four hours after treatment, Mindy's eyes focused for the first time. They were full of life. She was actively looking all over the place. Within a few days, after we had returned home, for the first time she was sucking her bottle. For me, this is a big step, because it means I no longer have to make her drink spoon by spoon. Now she drinks from her bottle like a pro.

Later, Mindy's mother added:

Mindy's improvements just continue to get better and better. She now smiles a lot on her own, which is so great to see, and when we call her she'll turn toward the sound of our voices.

Last month, for the first time, she started saying "Mama." I was in tears the first time she said it, and even now when she says "Mama" I still shed tears—tears of joy.

The most remarkable news is that we recently took Mindy to get a SPEC scan of her brain. The 3-D reconstruction showed that there was a marked increase in the size of the cortex of Mindy's brain, compared to her previous SPEC scans. (This is medical diagnostic proof of actual brain growth).

I'd like to let other parents with children who have disabilities like my daughter know that they should never give up hope. Follow your heart, and if people speak to you negatively and say there is nothing that can be done, just do your own homework and make your own decisions.

I just followed my instincts and my heart. If I hadn't, I would not have learned of the fetal stem cells, and Mindy would not be making any of the improvements she continues to make now.

Ian

Ian was 29 years old when he came to me from Australia. He had lived with cerebral palsy all his life. Doctor after doctor had told him that nothing could be done to help him.

Ian's condition had left him confined to a wheelchair, his limbs contorted. He experienced frequent, uncontrollable shaking in his arms and legs. He was extremely sensitive to cold, which made his limbs shake all the more. He would sit in his wheelchair slumped and bent over, his head turned to one side in spasm.

It was extremely difficult to understand what Ian was saying because of his slurred speech. He drooled constantly, had difficulty swallowing, and he would thrust his tongue out of his mouth constantly and involuntarily.

I have grown to love and deeply respect Ian because despite all his difficulties, he has maintained an exceptionally positive attitude. He enjoys writing, despite the difficulty of using a pointer attached to his head to peck out one letter at a time on a keyboard. He has kept a detailed record of his journey since he began receiving fetal stem cell therapy. Here are excerpts from his journal over the first year following his first treatment.

As soon as the stem cells were injected, my swallowing became much easier and it is much less difficult to move my legs.

My drooling has completely stopped and my tongue control is perfect.

My body has never felt so relaxed.

The shaking in my legs is almost nonexistent. I am now able to bend down and touch my feet and then can sit back up again, something I was completely unable to do.

Many people are commenting on how much my speech is improving and more and more people are starting to be able to understand me.

My feet were always cold, now they are warming up. Dad commented on how my muscles seem to be stronger.

My bowel function is much better. I used to be constipated, having a bowel movement only every three or four days, but now it's every day.

The shaking in my legs has ceased completely.

Ian chose to receive a second fetal stem cell treatment the following year. Here are some excerpts from his journal over the following few years:

While Dad was putting me to bed, I slipped while I was standing up, but I took a step and was able to stop myself from falling. Unbelievable!

This is one of the best improvements so far. You'll be very pleased to know that I'm now able to take 31 steps. The strength in my body is unbelievable. Week by week, I am getting stronger, and I know that it is the cells that are doing their job.

Today I was able to bite corn off the cob for the first time ever!

I have some fantastic news. Last week, I went to the osteopath for the first time since I've started the fetal stem cell treatment and his first comment was, "A lot of the excessive tone in your muscles has gone. I don't know of any treatment or method that can fix high tone."

Got into the pool today and did not feel cold at all, even after being in the water for one hour!

I am able to play a racing game on the PlayStation. The game consists of controlling a steering wheel and using foot pedals. This is incredible, considering my condition before I first received the stem cells.

My body has never felt so relaxed, like it is now. I feel completely different than from before the fetal stem cells. I feel more "normal" if that makes any sense.

The degree and nature of positive changes in the patients you have just read about has never before been reported within a group of cerebral palsy patients.

I feel it bears repeating that, because of the established attitudes toward fetal stem cell therapy and prohibition of its use, thousands of children and adults are denied a vastly improved quality of life and are therefore condemned to remain prisoners within their own bodies.

Cirrhosis

Cirrhosis of the liver is a slowly progressing disease which scar tissue replaces healthy tissues. As the scar tissue becomes more abundant in the liver it interrupts normal function and the normal blood flow through the liver and the functions of the liver can no longer appropriately take place

According to the National Institutes of Health (NIH) cirrhosis of the liver is the 12th leading cause of death in the United States.

The diseases that lead to cirrhosis do so because they injure and kill liver cells and the inflammation and repair that is associated with the dying liver cells causes scar tissue to develop.

Alcohol consumption is the most common cause of cirrhosis, particularly in the Western world. The development of cirrhosis depends upon the amount and regularity of alcohol intake. Chronic, high levels of alcohol consumption injure liver cells. Thirty percent of individuals who drink daily at least eight to sixteen ounces of hard liquor or the equivalent for fifteen or more years will develop cirrhosis.

Other common causes of cirrhosis are viral hepatitis B and C.

According to the present medical wisdom, liver damage from cirrhosis cannot be reversed.

When cirrhosis is far advanced, liver transplantation often is the only option for treatment.

I have treated one patient for cirrhosis. The following is a letter I received from him post treatment with the fetal stem cells.

Here is a summary of my liver disease, before and after the fetal stem cell treatment.

By William C. Rader, MD

My problem was cirrhosis of the liver. I promised myself and God that if your treatment worked I would become a better person. My liver disease was so bad that I was told by the doctors I would die if I did not get a liver transplant very soon, so they put me on the liver transplant list. It was about that time that my pancreas and gallbladder also began to shut down. I was told it was very unusual to see all three organs go down at the same time.

Sy *I suffered a 50-pound weight loss and had trouble thinking and remembering things. My skin and eyes became very jaundiced. I had severe fatigue, a stomach ulcer, and could not at all perform sexually.*

Toxic Liver

I considered myself a dead man.

Then came my treatment with the stem cells. It may sound crazy, but I could feel positive changes happening inside in only two days.

After three months, my liver was significantly better, to the point where I was taken off the liver transplant list, and my pancreas and gall bladder were basically fine. My stomach ulcer was gone, my mind was clear again, and I was also able to have a normal sex life.

It now has been six months since I received the stem cells. I weighed 120 pounds before treatment and now I am back to my normal weight of 166 pounds. All my liver tests are normal. My Hepatologist and Hematologist shake their heads in disbelief. After reading my lab tests one of the doctors actually said "I can't believe this shit you're not even supposed to be alive". None of them is willing to go on record that I'm a living miracle but I am.

All my friends and family who tried to talk me out of getting the stem cells are now applauding my success. I'm a poster child for you Dr. Rader.

262

Cirrhosis

It has almost been one and a half years since I started to recognize that I am an alcoholic. I'm proud to say I have been clean and sober for the past 15 months!

Coma

A coma is an extended period of unconsciousness from which a person cannot be revived, even with the most extreme stimuli. Coma itself is not a disease; it is a symptom of a disease or a response to an event like a head injury, which is the most common cause of coma.

During coma, patients—although alive—cannot move or respond to their environment. The responsiveness of the brain decreases as the coma deepens, and when coma becomes very severe, important reflexes such as breathing are lost, and the patient will die unless placed on life support.

Certain cases of coma can result in a persistent vegetative state, a condition in which the patient remains bereft of thought and awareness indefinitely. In this condition, patients may make spontaneous movements, and their eyes may even open in response to external stimuli, but they are unable to speak or respond to verbal cues or to their environment.

The outcome for a patient in a coma or persistent vegetative state depends on the location, severity, and extent of the brain damage. Outcomes can range anywhere from the rare full recovery to death.

More commonly, patients who do emerge from a coma can have a combination of physical, intellectual, and psychological deficits. Sometimes a coma patient will remain in a vegetative state for years, even decades. In such cases, no known medical intervention can reverse the process, and the best that conventional medicine can offer is ongoing life support, accompanied by the watchful waiting of the patient's loved ones.

I have used fetal stem cell therapy for patients in various stages of coma. The fetal stem cells helped the patients achieve a level of recovery that their primary physicians had considered beyond reach.

I have observed varying degrees of recovery in my patients, ranging from being taken off life support to completely emerging from the coma and returning to a relatively normal state.

Harry

Up until he was seven, Harry had been a perfectly normal child. Then, suddenly and inexplicably, Harry fell into a coma. Although his parents took him to top specialists at many medical centers, they all failed to provide a definite diagnosis; they were unable able to see on his MRI why a portion of his brain had become damaged. Harry was diagnosed with various diseases, ranging from herpes simplex encephalitis to tuberculoses meningitis. But the diagnoses turned out to be mere speculations that could not be proven.

Still to this day, unable to determine the cause of his brain damage, each of his doctors gave Harry' parents a very somber prognosis.

When I met Harry, his movements were random, and he could not respond to any specific stimuli. His arms and legs jerked spasmodically, he appeared to be in a constant state of muscular tension, and his eyes were unable to tear.

Although he did have a gag reflex and could swallow liquids, to achieve proper nourishment he needed to be fed through a feeding tube surgically implanted in his stomach.

Coma

One month after his fetal stem cell treatment, his mother sent me the following progress report:

Harry is more relaxed, and his muscles do not tense up nearly as often. And if they do, it only lasts for a short time. He is now able to tear, he is making noises such as murmuring and sighing, and he yells appropriately if he's in pain. He's able to eat solid food for the first time. He's also able to concentrate on light, especially shadows on the ceiling. His stools are now solid and regular. When we lay him on his front, he struggles to pick his head up. In general, he is more aware and comfortable. For the first time, we now have hope. My husband and I feel our son is beginning to return to us.

Three months later, Harry's mother wrote:

Harry had a follow-up MRI for comparison with his pre–fetal stem cell MRIs. His neurosurgeon said that he had never seen anything like this before. He told me that Harry's MRI was completely different, and that not only has the area of Harry's brain which was damaged gotten smaller, but he actually now has new brain growth.

Originally they told me that Harry was completely brain damaged and that he would never come back in any way. Also they said there was nobody out there who could offer me any help.

Harry is now eating through his mouth, so we were able to remove his feeding tube. Nobody thought this could ever happen.

He is so relaxed and he has no spasms at all. His pupils are smaller, and his eyes move together. He even looks normal, and you wouldn't think that there was anything wrong with him.

Harry received tens of millions of the pluripotent fetal stem cells, which have the innate ability to become any of the 220 type of cells in the human body, as well as tens of millions of pure neuronal stem cells.

They know where to go and what needs to be "fixed", which is why Harry's fetal stem cell treatment resulted in a positive outcome, even though his doctors were unable to diagnose the cause of his brain damage, which resulted in his coma.

Remember Jake from an earlier chapter? Five-year-old Jake had a rare brain infection, suffered a series of debilitating strokes, and was left in a semi-vegetative state severely brain damaged.

Sixty days after his stem cell treatment, Jake "woke up."

And here is the fascinating part: He knew the names of the nurses caring for him—nurses he had never met before his hospitalization. He also knew the names of their husbands and boy-friends, because he heard them talking to them on the phone.

Jake's case illustrates the importance of relating to loved ones in coma as if, at some level, they are cognizant of our presence.

My limited experience in the treatment of coma patients indicates that people in coma have far more awareness than previously thought. Spending time with them—talking, touching and relating as you normally did before—can help move a patient toward consciousness, as opposed to their sinking deeper and deeper into their coma.

Cystic Fibrosis

About 30,000 people in the United States are afflicted with cystic fibrosis. It is a life-threatening genetic disease that mainly affects the airways in the lungs and the digestive system—the stomach, intestines, and colon.

Cystic fibrosis involves abnormalities in the chemical properties of mucus, causing it to be thicker than normal in consistency.

In the respiratory system, the abnormal mucus obstructs airways, making it difficult to breathe. The thick mucus also leads to repeated multiple lung infections.

In the digestive system, abnormal mucus can obstruct ducts in the organs involved in digestion. They suffer from malabsorbtion syndrome, making it difficult for patients to digest food and thus absorb nutrients.

According to a recent report by the Mayo Clinic, cystic fibrosis has *no known cure*.

Although I have had the opportunity to treat only one patient with cystic fibrosis, I include it here because of its importance.

The case history is summarized in a letter I received from the patient's father.

Charles

Dear Dr. Rader,

As you know our son Charles was diagnosed with cystic fibrosis as an infant; throughout the past 16 years we have made every attempt possible to provide our son with a healthier life.

In early January Charles's health began to weaken again and he began to get fevers and infections. Over the next few months the situation became worse than it had ever happened before. New and dangerous infections started to emerge. At one point during this nerve-racking experience Charles had developed sudamonus and staph pneumonia.

On April 14 Charles was admitted into the intensive care unit. I told the infectious disease doctor that we were planning on getting Charles treated with fetal stem cells. She became very upset and accused us of doing something very dangerous that could seriously harm our son and refused to discharge Charles from the hospital, if he was to receive the fetal stem cells. We told her Charles was our son and we were going to do what we felt was best for him. The doctor then attempted some political maneuvering with the hospital's attorney to stop us. After several days of haggling, we were finally allowed to have Charles discharged, if we signed a document that it was "against medical advice."

The next day, still on continuous oxygen, we took Charles to you to receive the fetal cells. Within one hour of having the procedure done, Charles did not require his oxygen tank and he started to feel much better.

Due to the high doses of antibiotics that were given to Charles prior to having the treatment done, he developed diabetes, needing up to 15 doses of insulin a day. After the treatment his blood sugar levels began to decrease.

My wife and I were in disbelief of the improvements Charles had made in such a short period of time.

Ironically, two weeks after we signed out of the hospital, we received a message advising us to return to the hospital stating: Charles was in his last stages of the disease.

40 days after he was treated, we were able to completely stop giving Charles shots of insulin. Charles's energy, strength and weight began to increase. At this point he weighed approximately 87 pounds in contrast with the 80 pounds he weighed before the treatment. Charles had picked up his golf clubs which hadn't been done in a very long time and he was back at the driving range!

Approximately 2 weeks later, Charles's fever and coughing stopped. During this time we had him on two very mild antibiotics.

For my daughter's birthday, she requested we go to Big Bear for the day. We were very hesitant to bring Charles, being it is close to an elevation of over 6700 feet. He told us he felt strong enough to go, so we did and he was fine.

We took Charles for a checkup 2 months after his treatment. All the doctors were blown away by his recovery. He received 12 blood cultures and one sputum culture; everything came back negative except for a mild form of sudamonus. They gave us a routine antibiotic, which he was to take once a day.

3 months after treatment Charles's weight went up to 106 pounds and he continued to be more and more energetic. Approximately at the 6 month post treatment, Charles played in a golf tournament at the Lake Arrowhead country club where he obtained a one over par coming in 4th place.

I can proudly say I have my fun, loving, energetic son back after months of agonizing doubt.

Charles is doing superb. At the moment he is diligently practicing hard, confidently waiting for his chance to compete as a professional golfer.

Without this glorious opportunity and newly founded technology I do not know how our lives would be at this present time. My family and I would like to thank you from the bottom of our hearts for helping my son live a healthier happier life.

In my heart and soul I know this treatment saved my son's life.

These described changes occurred after administering the fetal stem cells to an "untreatable" teenager, in his "final stages."

Down Syndrome

Down syndrome is the most common genetic cause of severe learning disabilities in children, occurring in 1 in every 700 to 800 infants. It causes lifelong mental retardation, developmental delays, distinct physical malformations, and other problems.

According to the Mayo Clinic, Down syndrome cannot be cured.

The chance that a woman will give birth to a child with Down syndrome increases with age because older eggs have a greater risk of improper chromosome division. At age 35, the risk that a woman will conceive a child with Down syndrome is 1 in 400. By age 45, that risk increases dramatically to 1 in 35.

Cells normally contain 23 *pairs* of chromosomes—Children with Down syndrome have *three* copies of chromosome 21, rather than the normal two copies (a condition called trisomy 21).

Children with Down syndrome have a distinct facial appearance, including most or all of the following: flattened facial features, protruding tongue, small head, upward-slanting eyes, and unusually shaped ears. They also tend to have poor muscle tone and broad, short hands with relatively short fingers.

Chris

Chris was brought to me when he was seven months old. His blood test was positive for trisomy 21, Down syndrome and he exhibited all of the symptoms described above.

As Chris was the first Down syndrome child brought to me for treatment, I explained to his parents that I thought fetal stem cells could help but I couldn't say definitively that they would. After much deliberation, they decided to go ahead with the treatment.

Within the first year following treatment, all his symptoms *reversed to normal.*

- His face, the bridge of his nose, and his forehead all became rounded.
- His tongue no longer protruded.
- His head grew to normal proportion.
- His eyes became parallel.
- His ears grew to the proper size and position.
- He gained normal muscle tone.
- His hands and fingers became normal in shape and size.

Perhaps most important was the news from a pediatric neurologist specializing in Down syndrome to whom Chris was taken for evaluation. Not only did that doctor's report validate all the physical changes I have noted; she also found *Chris's IQ to be higher than normal* for his age.

She told his parents: "If I did not know he was a child with Down syndrome, I never would have guessed it."

Chris's case is yet another successful result of fetal stem cell therapy that has *never occurred before in the annals of medicine.*

Since Chris, I have treated more children with Down syndrome. Chris, being the youngest, had the most dramatic results, but the other children—ranging from four to eight—also experienced significant positive changes.

Down Syndrome

One other note about Down syndrome: it is common for pregnant women in their mid-thirties or older to undergo amniocentesis testing for the presence of trisomy 21, the genetic defect causing Down syndrome. In some cases, when test results are positive for trisomy 21, women choose to abort their pregnancies. I think it might be possible to negate this defect by injecting fetal stem cells directly into the amniotic fluid of a woman carrying a Down syndrome fetus, thereby eliminating the choice of abortion.

Eliminate Bone Marrow Donor Registries

The use of Fetal Stem Cells completely eliminates the need for Bone Marrow Registries, which in the United States alone keeps track of 4.5 million donors through the National Marrow Donor Program.

Donor matching depends on measurements of human leukocyte (white cell) antigens (HLA). A "perfect match" would be a donor whose marrow matches six out of six of these antigens. *HLA (WBC Antigens)*

But even with a perfect match, immunosuppressive drugs must be administered to help ensure that the donor cells would not fatally attack the patient (Graft versus Host Disease). *Rejection*

These immunosuppressive drugs severely lessen all immune function, and therefore leave the patient weak and susceptible to severe and at times even fatal infections.

Even under the best of conditions; a perfect match and the proper immunosupression an estimated 25 percent of patients will still die. *death Rate 25*

Stored in liquid nitrogen at my facilities today, are fetal stems cells, which due to their lack of a cellular fingerprint do not require the use of dangerous immunosuppressive drugs. They are readably available and can be used to save the lives of every bone marrow transplant candidate without having to wait until a match is found. Today all too many patients die, while waiting for their donor match.

There are other marked benefits with the use of the fetal cell.

After the normal bone marrow transplant procedure is performed, it usually takes 20 days in a "sterile clean room" for white blood cell counts (the immune system) to return to normal, leaving patients at significant risk of serious infections. But if the fetal stem cells are used, it takes only 3 to 5 days for the white blood cell count to return to normal levels.

*Today the average bone marrow transplant requires the use of *2 million* stem cells per kilogram of body weight. A bone marrow transplant using fetal stem cells requires only *25 thousand* fetal stem cells per kilogram of body weight; that's eighty times less the number of stem cells and they achieve a far superior overall outcome. Also the patient acquires a "new fetal" immune system that's at least ten times more powerful than that of a normal, healthy adult.

Even the cost of bone marrow transplants would significantly decrease if fetal stem cells were used.

Donor registries are maintained around the world to help support the ever burgeoning bone marrow transplant field. Using fetal stem cells these registries and their searchable databases are no longer needed, saving millions of dollars in costs as well as the personal sacrifice of untold numbers of donor volunteers.

Epilepsy

Epilepsy is a brain-function disorder that results in recurring seizures. It affects 5 to 10 out of every 1,000 people. Over two million people in the United States suffer from epileptic seizures, and modern medicine offers no help beyond attempting to manage their symptoms.

def The word "seizure" comes from Latin and means "to take possession of." That's exactly how many people who experience seizures describe them: as if something else has taken possession of their bodies.

During epileptic seizures, people often lose consciousness and/or control of their motor functions, which often results in convulsive, jerking muscular movements. Some epileptics are victims of a vicious cycle in which continuous, uncontrollable seizures cause increasing degrees of brain damage, which in turn worsens the frequency and severity of the next seizure.

In some cases, the seizures remain resistant to all anti-seizure medications. This is referred to as intractable epilepsy. I have successfully treated patients suffering from this severe, intractable form of epilepsy—most of whom had tried many other forms of therapy with little or no results.

Here are the stories of several of my epileptic patients.

Jennifer

Dear Dr. Rader,

Jennifer was born on May 16, 2007. She was diagnosed with epilepsy, microcephaly (abnormal smallness of the head), global delay, and static encephalopathy (abnormal brain structure). When we brought

Jen home from the hospital she was unable to swallow, blink, move appropriately, and was given a poor prognosis. We were told to prepare for the worse and that a children's home should be seriously considered. Since her birth Jen had been in and out of the hospital every 2-3 months for various infections. Her immune system was severely compromised and it was a struggle to move forward with the constant interruptions from illness.

On top of that in September 2007 Jen's seizures manifested as the worse kind; she was diagnosed with Infantile Spasms (IS) (an involuntary and abnormal muscle contraction)

Infantile Spasms were more than her little body could handle. She quickly began to deteriorate. Jen was becoming unaware of her surroundings and was unable to focus her eyes. She lost all motor control she did have and was slowly slipping away. She was on four different medications to control the seizures, but was still having 8-10 per day lasting from 5-20 minutes in duration. She was non-responsive, non-coherent, and rapidly progressing into a vegetative state.

We were watching our little girl die in front of us and we were being told that there was nothing we could do. But we were unwilling to give up.

After many hours of research we learned about Medra in January 2008. We knew that if she was going to have a chance to survive we had to try your stem cell.

Jen had her first stem cell treatment on March 28, 2008. As we drove back to the hotel from the first treatment, we began noticing changes. Jen's eyes were focused and she was looking around as if she woke up. As the next 12 days passed she began to have fewer seizures.

April 9, 2008 was the last seizure Jen had. She was off all seizure medications by August 2008.

Jens seizures were gone and she was awake. It was as if the lights were turned on again and she was back. After multiple specialists told us that there was nothing we could do to stop the Infantile Spasms; the stem cell therapy cured them with one treatment. We had our little girl back and she was fighting with all her strength to recover from everything that she had lost due to the IS.

Beyond the seizures going away and her responsiveness returning, we had hope. Hope that our little girl had a chance at life. Hope that stem cell therapy could give her so much more than what we could have ever imagined. Hope for a life full of experiences, joy, and love!

Jen returned in September 2008 for her second treatment. It was an amazing immune system boost. She went from September 2008 to January 2010 without even one infection. During that time she began making leaps in bounds with her cognition and movement.

Jen also had changes in her diagnostic testing. Her EEG, CT, & MRI had normalized, and her hearing test went from a "severe and profound" hearing loss to only a mild one.

She experienced an increase in her head growth and she no longer has the diagnosis of microcephaly!! Jen was also downgraded from having an active seizure disorder to a history of seizures. We were so excited, she had a chance at life, and we were now fighting for an increased quality of life.

We had a third treatment in September 2009; with the third treatment Jen has gained significant strength with her large muscle groups. With each treatment she gets stronger and progresses toward a different mile stone. By this point her specialist and therapist could no longer deny that stem cell therapy was responsible for playing the major role in her recovery and progress.

Without your foresight our daughter would not be here today. Thank you for playing such a huge part in saving her life and making the life she will have, full of joy and accomplishment. There are no words that can truly express the gratitude we feel. We only hope that watching Jen's progress gives you joy and you find fulfillment in the miracles you make possible for so many families. Thank you for saving our baby girl.

Aaron

Aaron was born a perfectly healthy baby and remained so until he received his first vaccination. A few hours after being immunized, he began to have four to five seizures a day of mild to moderate intensity.

Because of the timing of the vaccination and the onset of his seizures, his parents suspected that the vaccination had caused the problem. When their doctor's office contacted them to schedule a second vaccination, they decided to first meet with the doctor to express their concerns.

Aaron's parents explained to the doctor that they did not want Aaron to have the second vaccination. The doctor responded that failing to immunize their son would leave him at risk to severe, even fatal infection. After more urging by the doctor, his parents finally acquiesced, and Aaron received his second immunization.

Epilepsy

The next day Aaron's seizures increased from four or five a day to approximately 350, and continued at that rate every day thereafter. The seizures also increased in intensity.

At times he went into status epilepticus, an attack of many seizures in rapid succession, during which he stopped breathing. The oxygen deprivation caused by these repeated attacks caused Aaron to suffer ever increasing brain damage

The seizures were intractable; while some medications brought about minimal reduction in the frequency of the seizures, no medication could stop them. The seizures made it almost impossible for Aaron to sleep.

His amazing parents took turns watching over him and rocking him in their arms, in eight-hour shifts, 24 hours a day.

Eventually, Aaron's condition worsened to the point that his physician told his mother that nothing more could be done for him, and his survival was doubtful.

After many months of conversations with me, and after trying every other treatment they could find with no success, Aaron's parents went forward with fetal stem cell therapy.

Aaron was three years old when he was brought to me. A month after Aaron first received treatment, his mother wrote:

I have very exciting and wonderful news. Aaron's seizures have diminished to just about zero. He's gone from approximately 350 seizures a day to just a few, if any, each day, and those that he does have are not at all severe.

His sleeping pattern is much better as well. He is now able to sleep more each night without the constant waking-up pattern that my husband and I have battled for years.

A month later, Aaron's mother wrote me a second report:

All of Aaron's therapists are amazed at his progress. His sleep patterns continue to improve as well. Before Aaron received the stem cells, he would wake up very often during the night because of having a seizure in his sleep. Then, after the seizure passed, he would be unable to go back to sleep. Now, if he does awaken, he can easily be rocked or gently moved a little, and he will go right back to sleep. This is a real miracle to be able to see him beginning to sleep normally. It's a huge improvement.

In the past, Aaron would also have the most difficult time with his seizures when he was waking up. He would go into seizure for 15 to 20 minutes, and they were very intense. He would violently fling his head, arms, and legs. My husband and I were resigned to him doing so each time he awakened. We would try to allow him to go through this before we stimulated him too much, because that would only make his seizures worse. Now he is only twitching slightly when he wakes up and blinking his eyes a few times. This lasts for only a minute or two, and then he's done.

I have even been able to start weaning him off one of his seizure medications. We are weaning him very slowly, but expect to have him off all medications in the near future.

Overall, my darling boy is much more alert, smiling more, interacting more, using his eyes more, and has much better head control.

Several months later, Aaron was taken to his pediatrician for his annual evaluation. His mother wrote:

The doctor told me, "Aaron looks great!" He is now off of all medications. Previously the doctor had said to me, "Kids like Aaron never get better." He told me there was no need for us to bring Aaron back to him. I nearly cried in his office, since never before had a doctor told us that we didn't have to come back.

More exciting news. Today he got his new glasses. Pretty cool that he has glasses ... since his vision is coming back!!!!

The only way that his vision could be coming back is if that part of his brain is regenerating.

In 1998 after viewing the CT and MRI scans of Aaron's brain, the doctors at UCSF told us that the part of the brain that allowed for vision was destroyed-obliterated-gone... and that he would never see.

By William C. Rader, MD

Glasses are an amazing and wonderful thing to see on his face!

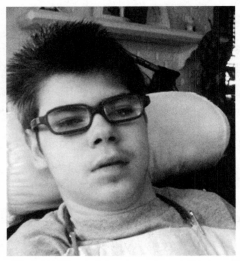

Finally, objective proof of the repair of my son's brain.
It's like a miracle!!

Carol

When her parents brought her to me, Carol was six and had suffered from epilepsy since she was a few months old. She was on several seizure medications. Due to the effects of her seizures, she had poor cognitive abilities, limited ability to follow instructions, trouble sitting still, and poor eating habits. Carol rarely interacted with her brother, and when she did it would often be in the form of aggression.

Three months after Carol's treatment, her mother wrote me this progress report:

The effects of the stem cells have given us new hope. Carol's cognition has noticeably improved. She is listening and responding to others better and able to follow instructions much like any other normal healthy child. She's also able to sit still and wait patiently when she has to, something that she could never manage before. Her appetite has noticeably improved. Since she received the stem cells, she has also begun playing appropriately with her brother, and overall she is acting more mature.

Carol's neurologist not only confirmed the positive changes we have seen in Carol, but said that they were "obvious and dramatic." He decided that it was no longer necessary for Carol to be on her seizure medication, so now she is off all of her medication.

Since then, though Carol still experiences an occasional seizure from time to time, they are far less in number and much reduced in their severity, to the point where they are almost unnoticeable.

After all that we have endured trying to get help for Carol, I can say without any hesitation that it is the fetal stem cells that have made such a difference. With everything else we tried, the benefits were minimal at best, and fleeting.

Steven

Steven was three years old when I met him. From the time he was five months old, Steven had suffered from Lennox-Gastaut syndrome, one of the most severe and intractable form of epilepsy. At times Steven suffered the rapid, successive seizures called status epilepticus, in which he was unable to breathe. This caused a progressive and unremitting increased level of brain damage. When Steven suffered a seizure, his parents could only watch helplessly. They were unable to stop the seizures, no matter what they tried.

By William C. Rader, MD

According to his mother:

Steven has had every medical test imaginable including EEGs, CAT, MEG, and PET scans, MRIs, blood work-ups, and genetic and metabolic tests, none of which has shown any structural or chemical cause for Steven's severe and intractable epilepsy.

Due to his Lennox-Gastaut syndrome, by the time Steven was nine months old he lost the ability to make noise, express emotions, and even cry. He became silent and withdrawn. He lost muscle control throughout his body, and could not eat for weeks at a time. He also was not able to have bowel movements on his own.

Last year, he had to be hospitalized one week out of each month for nutritional support.

Cognitively, Steven eventually regressed to the level of a three-month-old child. After exhausting all the neurological experts at Children's Hospital, UCLA, and the NYU Medical Centers, and after trying 13 different anticonvulsive drugs, the ketogenic diet, the surgically implanted Vagal nerve stimulator, osteopathy, homeopathy, and acupuncture, we still had to stand by and watch Steven degenerate after a storm of seizures—30 to 40 seizures on a good, normal day, and seizures every three to six minutes on bad days.

Steven's parents contacted every stem cell therapy researcher they could locate, but these researchers were still experimenting on mice and offered the distraught parents nothing but vague predictions of future benefits to humans.

Epilepsy

Steven's mother and father communicated with me for over a year, asking many sophisticated, detailed questions.

His mother later wrote:

At first we were reluctant to pursue this treatment, given the lack of available data about the procedure. We were eventually persuaded by stories from other patients who understood our struggle first-hand and although their child's diagnosis wasn't necessarily the same as Stevens, they described miraculous recoveries in their children.

Steven was treated with fetal stem cells in July 2004. Seven weeks later, he was examined by his neurologist.

In a progress report following the examination, his mother wrote the following:

We had seen the neurologist one week before Steven was treated with the stem cells, and he was not too pleased that we were going to do the treatment. He told us it was a foolish waste of our money and was potentially dangerous.

After seeing Steven, the neurologist was speechless. He could not believe his multiple and marked improvements. Previously he had told us that Steven would only continue to get worse, but he still would continue to see him regularly in order to monitor him. Now he is stunned, speechless, and practically frantic because he is so excited. He told us that he cannot believe his eyes.

Three months after his treatment, Steven's father wrote of his son's progress to a friend and sent a copy of the letter to me:

Within a week after Steven was treated, we saw major changes. Now, three months later, his seizures are drastically reduced in type, frequency, and intensity. He averages zero to five per day.

Steven has gained incredible muscle strength and balance. He is also completely engaged visually, and he eats with a great appetite. He is able to have normal bowel movements, which continue to become more regular.

Best of all, his beautiful voice is back. He hadn't made a sound for two and a half years! While he still has a long way to go, we are watching him getting stronger and more engaged every day. His neurologist and physical therapists are awestruck by his daily progress. His physical therapists have noticed greater muscle control in his legs, back, arms, and neck. He's also been able to participate in physical therapy with less help from his therapists and is now attempting to take steps in his walker.

We are amazed and ecstatic, and more hopeful now about Steven's future than we have ever been. Still, we are frustrated that we waited so long before discovering this treatment and that so many other children and families do not have access to the treatment that is giving us back our son.

At the end of 2004, Steven received a second fetal stem cell treatment. A week later, his mother wrote me the following letter:

It's amazing how quickly we noticed the changes in our wonderful boy. Now, after his second treatment, he wakes up making sounds and continues until the evening. It's been so exciting to call all of our family and friends and have them hear Steven on the phone. Since he was silent for two and a half years, it seems like he has a lot to say!

As for his cognition, it's apparent that he truly understands us more and wants to communicate his needs, likes, and dislikes to us. His seizures continue to reduce in number and intensity. And sometimes he is experiencing entirely seizure-free nights, something that has never happened in the past.

Now that he has received his second dose of fetal stem cells, Steven is even stronger and brighter, and my husband and I are at last having the opportunity to see our son thrive.

Giving him all the opportunities that we enjoy in our lives is our long-term goal, and the stem cells are helping to make that a reality.

Two months later, Steven's mother wrote me another report:

Well, our wishes are coming true. Steven has been seizure-free for the past 13 days, and we finally got his smile back! This morning he smiled when he saw his nurse and was smiling again all through the night. I even got a chuckle out of him. Can I just tell you how amazing that feels?

Steven can spend hours on the ground crawling and displaying the immensely improved strength in his arms, neck, and back. He is even trying to push himself up into a sitting position. He is still vocalizing nonstop from the time he wakes up in the morning until he goes to bed at night, and he is saying things that are more like familiar words every day. We are starting speech therapy today, so Steven will probably write the next letter himself, or at least dictate it.

He knows what he wants and how to coax it out of me. He can also sit unassisted for minutes at a time with his arms bearing his weight, which is something that he definitely could not do before. I can't tell you how happy (and exhausted) I am to have a happy three-year-old who is so special and amazing!

A recent electroencephalogram (EEG) reading revealed significant normalization of Steven's brainwave activity. As I write this chapter, Steven has been seizure-free for over four years. His mother writes:

On behalf of our entire family, my husband and I want to express our infinite gratitude for all that the fetal stem cells are doing for Steven. Not only did they save his life, they saved all of our lives!

❋ Despite all the success I have had in treating patients, I have consistently been met with entrenched resistance in my efforts to shake primary doctors out of their medical prejudices.

These physicians have observed positive results in their own patients that have never been reported before, anywhere. And yet I am unable to enlist their help in bringing fetal stem cell therapy into the medical mainstream.

The following exemplifies a shocking example of a doctor's indifference—and a sad illustration of some of the reasons for it.

Richard

Richard suffered from intractable epilepsy. He was under the care of a well-known, highly respected pediatric neurologist who was a leading professor at one of the foremost university hospitals in the United States.

She diligently attempted to treat Richard with every known treatment. Nothing worked in her attempt to stop the unremitting seizures, which caused progressive damage to Richards's brain.

Richard's parents described this pediatric neurologist as being very concerned about Richard and responsive to their needs as parents.

Eventually, because of Richard's rapid decline, she was forced to summon them into her office and then sympathetically tell them that their son had only months to live.

Although they had expected to receive this news someday, the moment of its arrival was devastating.

But Richard's parents refused to give up. Through their continued research, they learned about my work and brought their son to me.

Within a matter of weeks after treatment, two major changes started to occur. First, Richard's seizures became less frequent and intense and more importantly, Richard's brain damage began to reverse.

His parents kept the pediatric neurologist apprised of these changes. She was always responsive to their calls and interested in their updates on Richard's progress.

Eventually the seizures stopped completely—*an outcome that had never been seen in a child with Richard's diagnosis in the history of medicine.* Richard's mother waited all day to be sure the seizures had really stopped. That evening, no longer able to contain her excitement, she called Richard's neurologist and left her a message about the great news.

The next day, Richard's mother did not receive a call back. This was unusual, since Richard's doctor had always returned her calls promptly. The doctor neither accepted nor returned her repeated calls over the next five days.

At about that time, Richard's parents learned that their neurologist was scheduled to speak at an international conference on pediatric epilepsy. They decided to attend the conference and bring Richard with them. When the family entered the lecture hall, Richard in his father's arms, they saw their doctor seated at the speakers' table. When they attempted to approached her, she left her seat and disappeared behind the stage.

The keynote speaker, one of the foremost pediatric neurologists in the world, was about to speak. They decided to stay and listen.

Afterward, they approached the noted doctor, with his father holding Richard in his arms. Richard's mother began to tell him of Richard's remarkable, unheard-of recovery. This leading expert cut off the conversation by extending his arm outward as if to fend off a nuisance, exclaiming, "That's impossible!" and then he walked away.

Even though Richard's mother is one of the most intelligent, powerful, and determined women I have ever met, the eminent doctor's rebuff of her child's recovery, left her depressed for weeks. But finally her depression began to transform into anger and renewed determination.

She stepped up her attempts to confront Richard's neurologist by sitting in her office. The doctor finally relented and explained the reason for her behavior. She said that when she had received the news that Richard's seizures had stopped, she excitedly shared it with the entire pediatric neurology staff at her university hospital.

The other doctors warned her that any association whatsoever with fetal stem cells could result in great damage to both her career and the university. She went on to say that since she was nearing retirement she would not risk ruining the solid reputation she had enjoyed her entire career.

In the past year, I have treated two more of this doctor's patients who had the same diagnosis as Richard, and I have seen the same "impossible" results. These patients were referred to me not through a change of heart by the doctor, but thanks to the energetic activism of Richard's mother.

This doctor has now seen three miraculously recovered patients in her practice. Does she continue to tell other parents that there is nothing more that can be done and that their child will die?

I don't know. But I do know that I have never received a patient referral from her and that she remains unwilling to speak with me.

If political correctness is the overriding factor in medical decision making, then "where have all the Doctors gone"?

Heart Disease

Heart disease is the leading cause of death in the United States, killing [1 million annually] more than a million people annually. Once a person survives a heart attack, the likelihood that he or she will die from a second one increases more than fourfold.

In the past, cardiac problems affected more men than women, but recent statistics show that 52.3 percent of deaths caused by heart disease occur in women. The cost of treating heart disease in the United States exceeds $56 billion per year. cost

A significant benefit of fetal stem cell therapy is increased blood flow to the heart, which can help reverse the compromised blood supply caused by coronary artery disease.

The enormous benefits of fetal stem cells on the immune-system also have a significant effect on one's cardiovascular health.

✱ Medical science has recently identified inflammation (the body's response in its attempt to deal with a disease or illness) as a primary cause of cardiovascular damage. The tenfold boost in immune system strength one gets from fetal stem cells helps fight off infectious agents, reducing both inflammation and the risk of cardiovascular disease.

The remainder of this chapter is devoted to my use of fetal stem cells to help cardiac patients. I'll start with case histories involving my customary treatment using hematopoietic and neuronal fetal stem cells. Then I will describe my latest research on injecting fetal stem cells directly into the heart.

Linda

By William C. Rader, MD

Here is a letter from my patient Linda:

Dear Dr. Rader,

For over seven years I was suffering from multiple severe heart attacks and heart failure. I was told I had diffuse disease of the coronary vessels of my heart and due to the blockage, my heart was not able to get enough oxygen.

The doctors' first attempt to bring more blood to my heart was angioplasty, where they inserted a balloon in my coronary artery to push it open. It didn't work. Next they tried stents, placing tubes in my blood vessels to keep them open. Over time they kept putting in more of these stents, but all of the blood vessels eventually closed back off.

Each time I was hopeful that what they decided to do would work. Then came the letdown that it had failed.

I was becoming more and more frightened and depressed. My ability to participate in the world around me was becoming increasingly limited. I had always been a very active and social woman, and now I was essentially becoming a hermit—weak, in pain, short of breath, barely able to even get out of bed, and afraid to leave the house for fear of having another heart attack.

Then, as a last option, the cardiologists decided on a double coronary bypass surgery, where they would put two new blood vessels in my heart. I warily agreed.

After the procedure I initially had some improvement, but then the new vessels began to close off, and once again I was left in my previous condition. I was put on seven different medications, including

298

the frequent use of Lasix, a medication to help remove the water building up in my lungs.

Then one day my doctor sat me down and told me that he was sorry but there was nothing else that could be done. Here I was, a person who throughout my entire life had been known as a happy, intelligent, optimistic, outgoing, and active woman, and I had now become someone who was questioning whether life was even worth living.

Attempting to not let these thoughts get the best of me, I decided to search for nontraditional options to my dilemma. That is when I found you, Dr. Rader.

Almost immediately after my first infusion with the stem cells, I couldn't believe how much better I felt. For the first time in years I not only had energy but actual stamina. Within just a few weeks all my symptoms began to disappear.

As of today, I have an overall feeling of wellness. I am completely symptom and medication free. My internist and cardiologist remain completely amazed (to me they appear dumfounded in spite of the fact that they are aware of my stem cell treatment). After my last visit, the same doctor who told me that there was no hope now sat me down and said, "You have a very strong heart." His only follow-up request was an annual stress-test cardiogram.

I truly believe I could not have survived these past four years either physically or emotionally without your fetal stem cells. My family and I cannot thank you enough for all that you have done. Even today it still seems hard to believe that I am me again.

Alan

By William C. Rader, MD

Alan was 69 when I first met him, and he suffered from congestive heart failure. He was on various medications for his condition, but he was still unable to climb stairs; in fact, he could walk only a few yards before becoming short of breath and having chest pain.

Three months after Alan received fetal stem cells, he wrote:

I can now actually climb two flights of stairs without any difficulties, and I am able to go to the park and play with my grandchildren without losing my breath or even becoming tired. To be able to walk and play with them is my greatest pleasure, one that I feared I had lost forever before I received the fetal stem cells.

My latest ejection fraction (a measurement of heart function), was much better, indicating how improved my cardiac function is. My doctor told me he has never experienced a similar recovery to the one I am making.

Roger

When I met him, Roger was 80 years old and suffered from a condition in which the electrical signals that passed through his heart were interrupted, interfering with the heart's ability to contract properly. Like many patients with heart conditions, he had great difficulty walking any distance without becoming short of breath.

Four months after Robert received fetal stem cells, his cardiologist scheduled him to have an electrocardiogram (EKG), a test used to monitor the electrical signals of the heart. The results showed a 20 percent improvement in Roger's condition. His cardiologist considered this exceptional, since Roger's previous EKG tests had showed his condition to be consistently deteriorating.

Roger reported that his energy levels were much improved. He could now walk greater distances, while only on occasion experiencing minimal shortness of breath.

Sam

When Sam came to see me, he was 72 years old and had been diagnosed with congestive heart failure. He couldn't climb up even a few stairs without experiencing extreme shortness of breath. Previous attempts by his cardiologist to reverse or at least slow the progress of Sam's condition had yielded little success.

Six months after Sam received fetal stem cells, his wife sent me a follow-up progress report:

Since my husband received the cells I have noticed the following improvements in him.

Overall, Sam looks and feels much better and has much more energy and endurance. He can even walk up steps without losing his breath. His lips are no longer blue and his heart no longer pounds laboriously, like it used to.

There has also been a definite improvement in the color and tone of his skin. His face looks younger and the bags under his eyes are gone. Even his hair color has begun to change, turning from gray to a dark brown, and his hair has grown back in some places where he had lost it.

But, most importantly, his lab results confirm the major improvements in his heart function, since his treatment.

In short, the stem cells have given Sam a new lease on life, and he and I are both very pleased with his progress.

Ken

Ken is a very successful entrepreneur. He had been extremely physically active all his life, and every day he and his wife enjoyed long walks, regardless of the weather. He was also an avid skier. For Ken, the word "retirement" was anathema. Well into his 80s, he took an active part in the daily operations of his company.

All of that changed when he developed congestive heart failure.

When I met Ken, he was 89 years old. He told me he felt like a shadow of his former self, weak and unable to engage in the physical activities—both at work and play—that he had enjoyed for so many years.

Although he took diuretics to reduce his body's water content, along with heart medications, his legs remained severely swollen due to the fluid accumulation characteristic of congestive heart failure. Despite consultations with eminent physicians around the country, Ken's condition continued to deteriorate, and he became increasingly depressed.

Just a few months after his fetal stem cell treatment, Ken called me to say that he had lost nearly 20 pounds of fluid, and that his condition had "dramatically improved." He was back to overseeing his company full-time, and was once again taking long walks with his wife every day.

In a letter I received later, Ken's wife confirmed his improved vitality, telling me that he looked and felt much younger. His depression was gone and, about to turn 90, he was once more looking forward to life and sharing new adventures with her.

A New Method: Straight to the Heart

I have developed an experimental method for injecting fetal stem cells directly into the heart using a unique procedure. It is benign and in some ways similar to a routine angiogram performed in a cardiac catheterization laboratory.

Initially, we performed this experimental procedure on two patients, choosing two standard medical criteria for heart function to measure the results.

The first criterion was the New York Heart Association Functional Classification, often referred to by the association's acronym NYHA. This method of evaluation relies on simple observation to place patients in one of four categories based on the limitations their disease places on physical activity:

Class I: The patient has no symptoms or limitations on ordinary physical activity.

Class II: The patient's symptoms, such as shortness of breath or chest pain, are mild and activity is somewhat limited.

Class III: The patient experiences marked limitations on activity due to chest pain and/or fatigue, can walk only short distances, and is comfortable only at rest.

Class IV: The patient is usually bedbound and experiences symptoms even at rest.

Our second criterion was an ejection fraction test. "Cardiac ejection fraction" is the medical term for the percent of the heart's blood content that is pumped out with each heartbeat. A normal ejection fraction in an adult male is approximately 58 percent. *NORMAL EJECTION FRACTION*

The patients were evaluated and classified according to the NYHA scale both before the procedure and a week after. Ejection fractions were taken immediately before and thirty minutes after the procedure. The diagnoses, test results, and outcomes of the patients are given below.

Patient #1, male, age 60

Diagnosis—acute myocardial infarction with complete blockage of the right coronary artery with a dilated left ventricle (that is, he had suffered a heart attack due to a blockage in the oxygen-carrying coronary arteries and had an enlarged heart).

Symptoms—extreme shortness of breath and chest pain after minimal exertion. Patient is essentially housebound.

Previous treatment—patient received all that modern medicine had to offer from his cardiologist.

Metrics prior to fetal stem cell treatment:
- NYHA **Class III**
- Ejection fraction **45%**

Metrics following fetal stem cell treatment:

- NYHA improved to **Class I** within one week.
- Ejection fraction **61%**—which is normal and represents a *35% increase in heart function within 30 minutes.*

Clinical evaluation—the patient completely returned to an age-appropriate lifestyle and remains so today (more than two years has passed since the procedure).

Patient #2, male, age 41

Diagnosis—accentuated (60%) left ventricle cardiomegaly of unknown etiology, with clean coronary arteries (that is, 60% enlargement of the left side of the heart for an unknown reason, with no restriction of the blood flow to the heart).

Symptoms—extreme shortness of breath and chest pain after minimal exertion. Patient no longer able to work and is essentially housebound.

Previous treatment—patient received all that modern medicine had to offer from a university-based cardiologist.

Metrics prior to fetal stem cell treatment:
- NYHA **Class III**
- Ejection fraction **32%**

Metrics following fetal stem cell treatment:
- NYHA improved to **Class I** within one week.
- Ejection fraction **59%**—which is normal and represents an *85% increase in heart function within 30 minutes.*

Clinical evaluation—the patient returned to work and has resumed his life as a fully functioning husband and father for two years as of this writing. A recent radiographic evaluation indicated his heart, once 60 percent enlarged, *is now normal in size.*

The outcomes achieved for these two patients, as measured, *have never before occurred in the history of medicine.*

Although a cardiologist would most probably view the above as impossible. I submit to you the following as "proof of concept." I have added in italics comparisons between the iPS cells and the fetal stem cells.

According to an article in the journal Circulation. (July 2009).

In a **mouse** study by the Mayo Clinic, investigators demonstrated that induced pluripotent stem (iPS) cells can be used to treat heart disease. The iPS cells are stem cells converted from adult cells. *(As I mentioned previously the potential for unexpected genetic modifications such as cancer exists in the iPS cells and is nonexistent in the fetal cell.)*

A heart attack was created in two groups of mice resulting in damage to their hearts. Two weeks later in the first group of mice and four weeks after the heart attack in the second group the iPS cells were transplanted into the damaged mouse hearts. *(My patients were treated not weeks but instead years after their heart attacks.)*

306

The investigators reported the iPS cells significantly contributed to improved structure and function of the damaged heart. They restored heart muscle performance lost after the heart attack, stopped progression of structural damage in the damaged heart and regenerated tissue at the site of the heart damage.

✗ The researchers concluded that using a person's own cells in the process eliminates the risk of rejection and the need for anti-rejection drugs. *(With the use of fetal stem cells there is no risk of rejection and therefore also no need for anti-rejection drugs).* One day this regenerative medicine strategy may alleviate the demand for organ transplantation limited by donor shortage. *(That day is already here)*

Timothy Nelson, M.D., Ph.D., first author on the Mayo Clinic study stated:

"This study establishes the real potential for using iPS cells in cardiac treatment."

Fetal stem cells are an actuality today in cardiac treatment not a potential based on mouse studies.

Recently, I ran into a well known Beverly Hills cardiologist whom I have known for many years. I told him the results that occurred and in what time frame, after my experimental intercardiac procedure.

His response was, "You know I have always had great respect for you, all these many years. Either you are the smartest scientist on the planet, or you are seriously deluded."

Since neither is true, I assume he was politely telling me the latter.

Infertility

An estimated one in every five couples in the United States are infertile. According to an investigative report by ABC News, attempts to conceive via assisted reproduction techniques used by fertility clinics have a 73 percent failure rate.

In men, infertility is primarily due to low sperm count. Several factors contribute to low sperm count, including chronic illness or infections, general poor health, poor diet, lack of exercise or excessive exercise, smoking, excessive alcohol consumption, fatigue, and stress. Elevated temperature in the testicles, which can be caused by habitually wearing underwear that is too tight, can also reduce sperm count. Other causes include blockages in the vessels through which the sperm travel and poor sperm motility.

A variety of factors can cause women to be infertile. Endocrine problems, such as irregularities in the adrenal, pituitary, or thyroid gland—which together help regulate a woman's menstrual cycle—can result in problems related to ovulation, the monthly release of eggs. Narrow or blocked fallopian tubes (through which the egg travels to reach the uterus) are another factor in female infertility. As with men, chronic illness, infection, stress, and poor diet can cause infertility. Additionally, some women produce antibodies that can damage or destroy their partners' sperm.

Medical practices for reversing infertility in women include in vitro fertilization, infertility drugs, hormone treatments, surgery, and induced ovulation. In men, the most common infertility treatments are hormone therapy and surgery.

Fetal stem cell therapy can be an effective, safe way to improving fertility. I have treated a number of patients, both male and female, who became fertile after they received fetal stem cells.

In fact, I counsel all of my patients, male and female—no matter why they have chosen fetal stem cell therapy—to take precautions against an unplanned pregnancy.

I have had cases in which the sperm counts of infertile men rose to normal levels after they received fetal stem cells. And I have seen women whose efforts to conceive had failed, despite trying many other treatments, able to conceive naturally following fetal stem cell treatment and give birth to normal, healthy babies. Furthermore, some of my female patients who had very recently begun menopause have reported the return of their menstrual cycles.

Here are two illustrative case histories:

Robert and Sheila

"Robert" and "Sheila" are fictitious names I have given to a famous and affluent couple. Because of their financial resources and influence, they were able to travel to major infertility clinics throughout the world. After exhausting all other options, they decided to try fetal stem cells.

In their case, it was Sheila who was infertile. Prior to receiving fetal stem cells, she had tried in vitro fertilization several times using state-of-the-art methods, but these procedures never resulted in a single fertilized egg. Two months after her fetal stem cell treatment, Sheila tried in vitro fertilization once again. Five out of eight of her eggs became fertilized. Nine months later, she delivered healthy twin girls.

That was five and a half years ago, and the twins remain perfectly healthy, normal children. According to their parents, "The girls are not merely normal, but extraordinary in all respects."

Allison

In her mid-40s, Allison received fetal stem cells as an anti-aging treatment. She disregarded my routine warning regarding a possible increase in fertility. After her treatment, she continued to engage in the rhythm method with her husband, which they had successfully used for many years.

Much to their surprise, Allison conceived and happily gave birth to a baby boy.

While it deserves only a passing mention, I have observed a curious trend in cases like Allison's in which women received fetal stem cells shortly before becoming pregnant. Their pediatricians have frequently remarked that the children are "off the scale" in terms of intellect and developmental abilities.

I cannot with any certainty attribute it to the fetal stem cells, but this phenomenon, if indeed it is one, I feel deserves further study.

Multiple Sclerosis

Approximately 400,000 people in the United States live with multiple sclerosis (MS), and each week 200 more are diagnosed. Multiple sclerosis is a progressive disease that affects the brain and spinal cord, resulting in losses in muscle control, vision, balance, sensation, and cognitive ability. MS is an autoimmune disease, meaning that the brain and spinal cord are damaged by their body's immune system, mistakenly attacking it as if their own normal tissues were a foreign invader.

The central nervous system controls body function via nerves that act as the body's messenger system. Nerves are covered by a fatty substance called myelin that insulates the nerves and helps transmit nerve impulses between the brain and other parts of the body.

MS gets its name from the buildup of scar tissue (sclerosis) in the brain and spinal cord. The scar tissues, called plaques, form when the myelin covering the nerves is destroyed—a process called demyelinization. Without the myelin, electrical signals transmitted throughout the brain and spinal cord are disrupted or cut off. The brain is left unable to send and receive messages to and from other areas of the body. It is this breakdown of communication that causes the symptoms of MS.

As an analogy, the myelin sheath is like the insulating material that surrounds an electrical wire. In both cases, the loss of the insulating material disrupts the transmission of the electrical signal.

The plaques and lesions of MS can be detected by MRI (magnetic resonance imaging), which allows the doctor to define the extent of the destruction and the progression of the disease.

Although steroids can help lessen the severity and frequency of MS symptoms and even, in some cases, slow the disease's progression, no cure for multiple sclerosis is currently known.

As this chapter will demonstrate, fetal stem cell therapy represents a significant advance in the treatment of multiple sclerosis, including remyelinization—the formation of new myelin on the nerves—evidenced by the disappearance of plaques in the brain and spinal cord, as seen on the MRI.

Here are some case histories, including several patients' own reports.

Arthur

When I met Arthur, he was confined to a wheelchair.

He suffered from very strong spasms that made it extremely difficult for him to straighten his legs, which were normally in a flexed position. On the first day of Arthur's treatment, I helped him straighten his legs, which required grasping his ankles, bracing my foot against his locked wheelchair, and pulling almost as hard as I could.

He had difficulty speaking and was no longer able to write.

All of this interfered dramatically with his ability to operate his business.

Within three months after receiving the stem cells, Arthur's spasms lessened significantly, not only to the point where he could straighten his legs on his own, but if someone steadied him, he could take a few steps. He also regained the ability to hold a pen and write.

According to Arthur, what was most important, the treatment enabled him to return to his work.

Carolyn

Carolyn, another MS patient, suffered from gait imbalance, extreme fatigue, heat sensitivity, and insomnia. Only three weeks after her fetal stem cell treatment, Carolyn wrote:

My gait and sense of balance have improved dramatically, and my sensitivity to heat has dramatically decreased. My stamina is greatly improved as well.

My improvements began almost immediately after I received the fetal stem cells. You'll recall that I could hardly walk. My gait was so bad that it looked like I was pedaling a bicycle, and my sense of balance was so off that I had to use a cane most of the time. I received the cells on a Friday. By Sunday, on my way back home from the clinic, I was trucking through the airport at a decent pace. I had no pain whatsoever, and my gait was relatively smooth and fast. I was actually able to walk on the moving walkway by myself without losing my balance, something I never could have done before!

Since returning home, my symptoms continue to get better and better. My energy levels and stamina get better every day, and my bowel movements are at last returning to normal. Prior to treatment, I may have had a bowel movement every three or four days. Now it's daily. That sure helps my attitude! The tremor that I had on my left side is also much improved.

Prior to treatment, I could not sleep through the night due to my pain and bladder urgency and frequency. I often went several nights in a row without sleeping at all. The very first night after my treatment, I slept well and straight through the night. This continues. I'm sleeping through each night, free of pain, and what's even better is that when I do have to get up I am able to go straight back to sleep, which enables me to wake up fully alert and well rested. Before, I remained in what I called a brain fog for a couple of hours after I got out of bed every morning.

One of the first symptoms of my MS, in fact the one that sent me to the doctor in the first place, was the fact that I had completely lost the ability to sweat. It got so bad that it became difficult to go outside during the summer long enough to get from the house to my air-conditioned car. I couldn't even take a hot shower! Now I'm sweating normally and able to tolerate the heat almost as well as I did before I became ill.

Another major improvement is the foot and right-hip pain that I lived with for many years. That pain dissipated within the first week after treatment, and within three weeks my feet and hip stopped hurting altogether.

A month later, Carolyn wrote:

I am continuing to experience improvements. I am cognitively much sharper. I continue to get up in the morning fully alert and wide awake. My libido has also increased, with a corresponding increase in my sexual pleasure, back to a pre-diagnosis level. My friends and family continue to comment on my obvious and significant improvements.

Barbara

Barbara's initial inquiry letter to Medra included this account of her symptoms:

Hello, my name is Barbara. I am 48 years old and was diagnosed with multiple sclerosis 12 years ago. My symptoms are waves of dizziness throughout the day, severe double vision, numbness in my hands and fingers, loss of sensation in my feet, and I drag my right leg when I walk.

I'm married. I have two teenage daughters and a dog that I would like to walk someday.

After her fetal stem cell treatment, Barbara wrote:

It has been a little over two months since I received the stem cells. During these past two months, I have noticed many significant changes. My gait has definitely significantly improved. The numbness in my fingers has decreased, and I can actually feel what I am grasping, and now I can wiggle my toes.

Another great improvement is that my double vision has markedly decreased. An added bonus, which I am not ashamed to say I love, is my "face lift." No more jowls and double chins! It is all up and tight, just like the rest of my body (breast and butt). I feel like Benjamin Button!

Julie

Recently I received the following letter:

Hello, Dr. Rader.

By William C. Rader, MD

It was so very nice to meet you and receive your treatment of fetal stem cells, for which I have been waiting and hoping for a very long time.

As I had told you, I was diagnosed with multiple sclerosis in 1994 after an initial, total left sided paresthesia (tingling of the skin). An MRI showed "many scattered foci of increased signal intensity", and a spinal fluid analysis showed oligoclonal bands (both of which are diagnostic criteria for MS).

I was admitted to the hospital for intravenous methylprednisolone (a steroid) therapy for five days, followed by tapering doses by mouth at home. I was able to recuperate in a peaceful environment on the family farm. It took me about a year to get 80 percent of the feeling back in my left side, during which time I had one migraine after another, continuing to this day, sometimes more and sometimes less.

I also experienced an inability to withstand cold—yes, cold. I know the norm for MS is an inability to withstand heat, but with me it's cold. It's as if I have a stainless steel rod for a spinal column, and my lower body has no circulation, no warmth.

For the last eight years my symptoms had been increasing. I was experiencing numbness, a deep aching and a humming vibrating feeling all throughout my body.

I was in chronic pain that kept me from enjoying any kind of life. Vicodin was the drug of choice to be prescribed, but due to the high risk of renal and or liver disease over prolonged use, I finally opted for a pain clinic that gave me methadone. I have been taking methadone for the last four to five years. It worked to some extent; however, it only took the edge off.

I was never able to sleep more than four hours at a time, making me a very irritable and worn-out person.

Prior to my treatment at your clinic last weekend, I stopped taking the methadone, wanting to be clean of medication and the effect it might have on my assessment of the fetal stem cell therapy I would receive. I am thrilled to report that just two hours after receiving the stem cells, upon returning to my hotel room, I experienced a lessening of the sensations I have had for the LAST DECADE.

I know this is NOT wishful thinking. I certainly have visualized, meditated, prayed, exercised, and followed Dr. Swank's MS diet to the letter. I have done myriad things trying to bring about self-healing over the years without any successful results.

Diet
For
MS

I am amazed to think some sort of re-mylenization (repair of the nerve insulation) has occurred so quickly, perhaps a thin coating that has subdued the majority of the pain in nerve endings?

I have guarded optimism, and yet I am embracing the moment as it is MINE. I couldn't even begin to express my happiness.

"Thank you" seems like empty words for such a dramatic change in my condition!

(Most probably the positive changes Julie experienced were a result of the "cytokine effect" as opposed to any kind of remylinization).

Doris

Doris was 46 when first treated with fetal stem cells. She had been diagnosed with MS three years prior.

By William C. Rader, MD

A month after her treatment, Doris wrote:

I am truly ecstatic with this healing process and the changes I am witnessing in my body!

The first thing I noticed immediately, during my flight home from the clinic, was that the always-present pain of spasticity and the pulled muscles in my body, especially in my neck and back, were completely gone. And they continue to be gone to this day. This had been a constant feature of my disease for well over three years. My legs are also becoming stronger. I find myself using my cane less and less.

Another positive change after I received the fetal stem cells was my lack of allergy and asthma symptoms during a weather period here in Los Angeles that normally would always cause me to have a severe allergic reaction. Now, four weeks later, I am still allergy- and asthma-free, which is phenomenal. My energy levels have also shot up tremendously, and I am not having the dizziness, confusion, spaced-out reactions and my mind and memory are improving.

Perhaps most amazing of all, I now find myself able to access levels of joy, passion, and faith that have been way beyond my reach for so many years.

A few months later, Doris wrote to me to report the results of her MRI:

Not only did the MRI show no new plaques, it also showed that some of the old plaques had disappeared. This is a huge positive difference. In the past my MRIs were horrible. I am at last moving in the right direction!

Having witnessed what I thought was impossible, I find myself crying tears of joy these last few days. I am eternally grateful for having discovered the stem cells and what they are doing for me!

Doris's case illustrates that we now have indisputable scientific proof (by MRI) that fetal stem cells can effect remyelinization of damaged nerve cells, with the subsequent disappearance of the plaques that are at the root of multiple sclerosis.

Not all the patients I have treated for Multiple Sclerosis have been as successful as the ones I have just described.

Some of my MS patients required multiple treatments before experiencing any significant benefit.

Muscular Dystrophy

Muscular dystrophy (MD) is an inherited disease in which muscle fibers are unusually susceptible to damage, initially resulting in muscle wasting and then eventually, the actual death of the muscle cell. Fat and connective tissue often replace the lost muscle fibers. This loss of muscle mass can be hard to see because the build-up of fat and connective tissue makes the muscle appear larger than it actually is.

Early signs and symptoms of Muscular Dystrophy include: weakness in the lower leg muscles, resulting in difficulty in running and jumping, difficulty in getting up from a lying or sitting position, frequent falls, a waddling gait, and in some cases, mild mental retardation. By late childhood, the children are eventually unable to walk.

Sadly, Duchene Muscular Dystrophy, the most common type, is terminal and death usually occurs before the age of 30.

Despite the fact that over 1.5 billion dollars have been raised for research by the Labor Day Jerry Lewis Telethon over the last 42 years, currently there is no cure or even a specific successful treatment for Muscular Dystrophy.

The following is a compilation of letters I received from the mother of a 4 year old boy with Muscular Dystrophy.

Dear Dr. Rader,

I am writing you to tell you Robbie is doing great. Starting immediately after his treatment, when we got back to the hotel room, he started going around in circles really fast which we have never seen him do before. Also at the hotel he climbed up about 30 stairs one foot after another like it was no problem, which was a shocker for us because he had an extremely hard time with stairs. In the past, he would have to hold on to the railing, to pull himself up the stairs. This time he didn't hold on to anything. He did it like a pro. He was so excited that when he got to the top of the stairs he started to clap and jump up and down yelling, "I did it mom, I did it mom."

That made me really cry because before we saw you, he was going right down hill. He couldn't do all the things that he is doing now. For the first time he was able to jump off the ground. He was so excited he kept doing it over and over. He is also starting to run which he never ever did and as the days go by, his running is getting better. He is trying to climb everything. I can't take my eyes off of him for a second. He has a thing with ladders which freaks me out. He can get into bed with no problem and is able to put on his pants on his own, which is a big deal for him.

Robbie's changes keep coming. His strength has really improved. He has a lot of strength in his legs now, which before were very weak. When he's sitting on the floor he used to use his hands on his knees to push himself up, but the last few weeks he just gets up like it is nothing. He has a regular gait and his calves are gone down to normal size, which before they were large.

Last Friday we took all the kids to the zoo which is over 700 acres. We rented a stroller for Robbie because, although he was much better, we were concerned he couldn't walk such a long distance. But that day he refused to get in the stroller and walked 6 hours! It was really amazing for us to see him having no problem at all walking that far.

His speech has significantly improved. He is now speaking in full sentences which he never did before.

Also, the treatment has really helped Robbie psychologically.

Robbie's attitude is very different from what it used to be. He has become very independent.

He is never sad, like he was before his treatment, because he couldn't do what the other kids were doing. Now he is confident, happy and always has a smile on that cute little face of his, which also makes us very happy.

Robbie went with us where there was dancing and for the first time in his life he was able to dance, he wouldn't stop, he just danced and danced. It was priceless.

The school called me to tell me everyone was amazed with the way Robbie came back to school. They see so much improvement in him, that he is really strong, full of energy and cannot be slowed down. He is also participating in gym which he didn't at all before and loves jumping on the trampoline.

About a week ago we awoke to a loud thumping noise, and discovered it was Robbie and his siblings running full tilt around the kitchen table, his running was incredible, better that we have ever seen before, it was very heart touching.

But strangely it hasn't all been roses. I am writing to tell you the stuff I have been through lately, but I look at my wonderful little boy and that makes it all better.

By William C. Rader, MD

The other day Robbie and I decided to take a walk and all of a sudden we were confronted by protesters on abortion, with pickets and signs. I guess they read about Robbie in the newspaper.

*When we tried to get away, they wouldn't let us pass and started yelling at me and my little Robbie, saying what we did is a sin against God and then one of them **spit on me**. I looked at them and said, look at my son, he was very sick and now he is healthy and then walked away with my head up high.*

It has been wonderful to sit back and watch how much he progresses every day.

I can truly say that the treatment has been a miracle for Robbie and we are so grateful to you for not only giving us this opportunity, but also free of charge.

We are so happy that Robbie has shown such great progress, because before we had to watch as he was continually going downhill and now since he got the stem cells, we are watching him rapidly going uphill. Every week we are seeing something new that happens or improves.

Robbie is easily doing things that before he either had a hard time doing, or wasn't even able to do. He is very funny. If you try to help him he gets really mad.

Everyday Robbie says that he loves you. He constantly tells us that Dr. Rader made his legs stronger and that he is all better.

We all have seen so much improvement in him it's crazy. You look at him and you would never know that he has muscular dystrophy, which of course makes us very happy and grateful we found you. It truly has been an amazing experience.

Larry was also 4 years old when his parents brought him to me for treatment.

Hello Dr. Rader,

My husband and I first want to say we are truly grateful and thankful for your caring and generosity.

After we were told the devastating news from our doctor that our son Larry had muscular dystrophy and although he said there was no real hope for recovery, we decided we were not going to give up.

Hundreds of hours of research later, my husband came across your Medra web site. This was our last hope, as Larry was unable to walk and his poor little legs were hard, stiff and very painful. And, so we called your office and scheduled the next available treatment.

Well five hours after treatment Larry walked up three stairs without holding on to anything or anyone. He has never done this in his entire life. It was so beautiful tears came to my eyes.

After we returned home Larry was still going strong. HE CAN WALK! He has only complained twice since treatment about his legs hurting him and this was only after walking two blocks. Also his energy level has gone way up.

Initially Larry surprised us with getting up from the floor, to a sitting position, without crawling to anything in order to pull himself up. He is also able to bend his legs more at the knee.

Early on post treatment he seemed to be aware and appreciate his newly found strength, as now he takes no business from his big sister.

He does think twice about hitting her; however this is great to see the fire and energy he has. I started to call him super boy.

Larry is now 16 weeks post stem cell procedure He has aquatic therapy every week. He is like a fish in the water. He is completely independent. He walks around in the pool without assistance. He has therapy 30 minutes as instructed and still wants more. His balance is excellent in the water. He can also float on his back without assistance.

Prior to the stem cell procedure Larry needed and sought assistance. Now he resents it if we try to help him. Larry's quality of life has improved so much. He has excellent self esteem and wants to try everything

We have had so much snow this year. He loves to walk around in it. His balance is great in the snow. Even on the icy areas he does well, and doesn't want assistance.

He skips, jumps on his trampoline, runs and has a good time. His level of activity has increased so much. Before the stem cells he was always tired and wanted to go to bed early. Now at night he doesn't want to go to bed he wants to continue to play. He likes to be on the go!

Today I received incredible news; Larry's CPK level dropped to ONE HALF of what it was 3 months ago. (CPK or creatine phosphokinase is an indicator of significant muscle wasting.) I had insisted that my doctor do another CPK test. He flat out refused and said it would be a waste of time and money, that it was done initially three months ago and it would only depress me because in a patient with muscular dystrophy it ALWAYS INCREASES over time. I finally was able to find another doctor who was willing to do the CPK test and look what happened. I am so excited that I am beside myself.

Muscular Dystrophy

This was an experience that was truly astounding. We met what I truly felt was one big family that really does care. In the past our experience with doctors was: we can only give him a pill for some relief of his symptoms. Sit back, wait and see and enjoy your limited time with him. The only course of therapy for Muscular dystrophy today is the steroid Prednisone with all of its negative side effects. In my heart I feel that stem cell therapy should be a CHOICE for families and patients with debilitating medical diseases.

Today, Larry has a chance at being a happy healthy little boy, and for this there are no words I can possibly say to you that could express our gratitude and gratefulness to you and your wonderful staff.

Parkinson's Disease

Unlike drugs, which work only fleetingly, until their chemical compounds are broken down, (stem cells)...can provide tiny factories...that work around the clock, producing the chemicals, hormones, and other molecules that our bodies need in order to function.

—Eve Herold, Stem Cell Wars

Each year, Parkinson's disease strikes 1 out of every 200 elderly people in the United States. The number of people suffering from Parkinson's is greater than the number of patients diagnosed with multiple sclerosis, muscular dystrophy, and Lou Gehrig's disease combined.

Parkinson's disease results from the lack of a chemical messenger, called dopamine, in the brain. This occurs when the specific brain cells that produce dopamine die or become impaired.

Parkinson's usually strikes individuals in their late middle age; the average age of onset is 60. However, the incidence of early-onset Parkinson's—in people younger than 40—has risen in recent years.

The disease seems to have a high genetic correlation. Between 15 and 20 percent of Parkinson's patients have a close relative who has experienced Parkinsonian symptoms, such as tremors.

Parkinson's is chronic and progressive, meaning its symptoms get worse over time. Typical early manifestations are slight trembling or shakiness in a hand, arm, or foot. As the disease progresses, it is characterized by slowness of movement, muscular rigidity, tremors, problems with speech, diminution of facial expression, shuffling gait, and defects in balance. Daily activities become increasingly difficult, and memory can also become impaired. In some cases, the patient becomes severely or completely incapacitated. There is no known cure.

The cost of Parkinson's disease in the United States exceeds $5.6 billion annually. The medications used to treat it are only palliative— intended to alleviate symptoms. These medications can lose their effectiveness over time, and they also have significant side effects. Ironically, over time, one of the side effects is to actually produce Parkinsonian like symptoms.

There is no known cure for Parkinson's disease.

Experts in the field of stem cell research have theorized that stem cell therapy might effectively treat Parkinson's disease, but with the stipulations that additional research is still needed and that successful treatment is probably 20 years away.

For over 15 years, I have treated Parkinson's patients. The degree of success I have observed, as with other illnesses discussed in this book, varies among individuals and with the stage of the disease. However, at a minimum, fetal stem cell therapy has effected a marked slowing of the progress of Parkinson's.

Typically my Parkinson's patients experience a reduction in their symptoms, and a number of them gained the pronounced results of the following case histories.

Victor

Victor is an attorney who formerly held elected political office. He had suffered from Parkinson's disease for 19 years before he consulted with me. In addition to the usual Parkinson's symptoms, Victor suffered from involuntary jerky movements called dyskinesia.

His condition had so deteriorated that he was confined to his bed and wheelchair and required full-time nursing care. He had to be helped in and out of bed; he could move on his own only by crawling.

Prior to seeing me, Victor had been told that his only remaining option was a surgical intervention called a pallidotomy. This operation involves drilling a hole in the patient's skull, then destroying specific areas of the brain in order to provide symptom relief. Pallidotomy does not offer a cure, but it is one of only a few treatments for Parkinson's available. (Others include drugs such as Levodopa and Sinemet, alternative medicines such as herbs, vitamins, and other supplements, and alternative treatments like acupuncture).

Fearing brain surgery, Victor kept putting off the operation. When he finally felt ready, his physician determined that his symptoms had advanced too far for him to be a candidate for the procedure.

With no other options left, Victor turned to his last hope: fetal stem cells. Despite the severity of his physical symptoms, Victor's mind remained sharp. I could see his intelligence in the questions he asked me during our initial conversations; his sense of humor was also very evident.

He arrived at the clinic in a wheelchair accompanied by his long-time nurse. On the day following his treatment, his symptoms began to diminish dramatically. Moreover, on that first day, Victor did something that astonished me and would certainly defy belief in the general medical community.

I went to visit him that day, as I do with all my patients, and found him in the lobby of his hotel, in his wheelchair attended by his nurse. I could see that his physical appearance had improved, and his speech was stronger and much clearer. The first thing he said to me was, "Sit in the wheelchair." When I asked him why, he repeated in a commanding tone, "Sit in the wheelchair." Then, to my amazement, with effort, Victor stood up from his wheelchair. Obeying, I sat down in the wheelchair. Victor grasped the wheelchair's handles for support and began to push me through the hotel lobby. He headed directly toward a group of hotel guests. I was sure Victor had lost control and that we were going to plow into these people. Instead, at the last moment, Victor turned away. He looked at me and began to laugh.

This is yet another demonstration of the almost immediate effects that cytokines can produce, even given the state of Victor's disease and the extent of his declining health.

In her last follow-up report, his nurse wrote:

Victor continues to walk, and the tremors in his hands, which previously were severe, have lessened significantly.

Victor's improvements are progressive and have never regressed, including his balance, gait, overall energy, general mobility, speech, and emotional well-being. His wit and sense of humor are at an all-time high.

Alan

Parkinson's Disease

Three weeks after Alan received fetal stem cell treatment for his Parkinson's disease, his wife Ellen sent the following report, summarizing her husband's medical history:

The earliest indication of Alan's illness was when he started complaining about being fatigued, and he was irritable—not at all his usual outgoing self. (He has always had a type-A personality). Within the next year, as he would get dressed for work, he would say, "I just don't know if I can make it today," but he would push himself and go. Then his left hand began to shake. Shortly thereafter, he was diagnosed with Parkinson's disease.

He became progressively worse over the next five years. Even though he was taking the maximum dosages of his Parkinson's medications, it did not help with his pain, rigidity, fatigue, discomfort, and sleep deprivation. Instead, as a side effect of all of his medications, he would have uncontrollable jerky movements of his face, tongue, and chest.

He began to shuffle instead of walk, his balance became very poor, and he was mumbling. I noticed that his right eyelid would sag or not open. His color was pale, and his face was almost totally expressionless.

He insisted on being left alone. Depression was taking over; he started talking about ending it all, saying that this kind of life was just unbearable.

Since Alan was raised a devout Catholic, I feel this was most significant of how much deterioration and suffering he was experiencing.

When I was finally able to get him to open up a little I realized how desperate he was, because he felt there was nowhere to turn for help.

When we left for the airport to receive the fetal stem cell treatment, it had been six years that he had been enduring his overwhelming symptoms. He could barely make it through the gates and to the plane. He refused to ask for help, and I do believe that numerous times he was nearly in tears. The worse his symptoms got that day, the more he tried to hide from me how bad off he really was.

To my amazement, the day after his treatment, when we arrived at the airport to go back home, he carried his luggage with no complaints; he was not shuffling, his balance improved, and despite our flight being delayed, he was in a better humor than I was. He told me, "Coming for treatment with all that walking was torturous. Now, going back home, I feel very strong. I have the energy I used to have."

We had a two and half hour layover, and he did great—even joking and talking to several people. By the time we finally arrived home, he was still going strong, and I was the one who was becoming short-tempered and tired.

When we finally got to our car, I couldn't wait to get home, but when we called our son, Alan told him we would stop by to say hi. I couldn't believe it; I was ready to fall into bed!

At the first sight of his father, our son just beamed. Without saying it out loud to each other, we were all afraid to think that the treatment could be showing such positive results that soon.

It's now been about three weeks since my husband received the cells. About a week ago, after Alan got out of the shower, he said, "I can now shampoo, tilting my head back with both my eyes closed, without *holding on to the handrail. I thought it would be impossible for me to ever be able to do that again."*

For the most part, each day is a new adventure. He's becoming more outgoing, more humorous, doing his funny little dance step. Everyone who sees him comments on the improvements in his gait, posture, voice, facial features, and how he is looking like his old self. Today he actually worked out with his brother, who is a weightlifter.

Alan still has some "off" times, but nothing like before.

To be honest, we are afraid to believe that things are improving so much and that it's for real, but you just can't ignore these incredible changes.

P.S. Alan is feeling AMOROUS again!

Andrea

Andrea, a writer, had suffered from Parkinson's for over five years before she came to me for treatment. Her body was stiff and her gait was noticeably unbalanced. She had chronic pain in her right shoulder and left hip, and hearing problems in her left ear due to what she described as "burbling" sounds inside her head. Her speech was so slow that at times understanding her was very difficult, and she was unable to control herself from continually drooling.

Andrea has always kept a personal journal, and she continued to do so after her initial fetal stem cell treatment.

The following are excerpts from her journal:

Day 1: Following a long flight back from the clinic, I wasn't even tired when I got home.

Week 1: Language facilitated. Much easier to talk. Takes less work. My right shoulder doesn't hurt; pain gone since the day I was treated. It is almost normally flexible. My left hip doesn't hurt either. Greatly improved and definitely more flexible. I can stretch in any direction and can bring my feet up more easily.

Week 2: My tongue works better. Feels normal, and it's easier to find the words I want to say. My left hip feels like something has been replaced. It is much more stable. My hearing is improving too. The feeling of fullness and the burbling sounds in my left ear are gone.

Week 3: It's clear that my balance is better. Every time I get up to walk, I'm surprised with the ease thereof. No feelings of achiness at all.

Week 4: I've stopped drooling and am able to leave my mouth closed instead of hanging open so much. I'm also producing more saliva for the process of chewing, rather than just salivating. And I can swallow with ease! It's almost normal. Everyone comments on my verve, energy, more balanced walk, more rapid and distinct speech, and mental acuity. It's very easy for me to think things through. They seem crystal clear. My typing is improved, and I'm beginning small dance steps.

Week 6: Today I actually went shopping on my own, for the first time in many, many months!

Week 7: My balance keeps improving. It's hard to believe, but I'm better off without my cane! Almost kept up with my daughter when we went walking. I do little dance steps and don't even fall.

Week 9: I am increasingly thrilled by the improvement in my balance. It's not totally normal yet, but has moved a long way in that direction.

Week 12: I find it easier and easier to dance. My massage therapist was astounded at the changes. She found that the mobility in my hips

338

improved from about 50 percent of normal to 95 percent. She was particularly astounded by the mobility in my right wrist. Previously there was essentially none. Now, it's suddenly quite normal

Week 15: This morning I could almost dance normally. If this keeps up, I'll be able to tango again!

Week 16: Yesterday I spent a lot of time on my feet cleaning out closets and drawers. I feel refreshed and my energy is restored, the way it used to be. Absolutely amazing!

Week 18: Today my massage therapist noted that the tension between my shoulders is completely gone. She described the area as being "like butter." Also, my therapeutic yoga instructor has been overwhelmed by my sudden flexibility and balance. As I performed the exercises she keeps saying, "Wow, wow!" My acupuncturist was also delighted with my ease of movement and commented that I had less edema.

Week 21: I am surprised at the ease with which I am catching up with my writing. Instead of being overwhelmed by too much pending work, it all seems so simple and straightforward. I have delightful fantasies about the next time I see my neurologist and he asks me to walk down the hall to show him my residual stability. I think I'll waltz!

Week 24: Recently I went to a friend's wedding. Everyone there who knew me was stunned by my improvement. One of my girlfriends said she couldn't believe how easily I was able to get into the car. It used to be tediously difficult for me to load myself into a sedan. Everyone told me, "You look wonderful. It's so good to see you looking like this!" A friend told me, "I've known you for five years now, and I have to say it was as if there were holes in your person, and now you are whole." My favorite moment was when another friend told me, "You are absolutely beautiful!"

Week 25: To my amazement, after at least three years of being unable to smell nearly anything, I am beginning to get whiffs of odors. When walking through a garden on a very warm day I could smell the flowers the whole time I was walking. This is something I hardly dared hoped for improvement on.

Week 26: Today I took great pleasure in demonstrating my newly re-established ability to dance the samba. My assistant's husband stopped by and stared at me, saying, "You look wonderful!" He told his wife later that I look ten years younger than I did a year ago. Let it be so!

Agnes

Agnes is a brilliant businesswoman who established a unique entertainment business that thrived for decades. Agnes was known for her creative instincts and for winning over Hollywood executives during business meetings with her intelligence, sharp wit, and ability to excite people about her ideas.

When Agnes developed Parkinson's disease, it severely impacted her business. Not only did she develop physical symptoms; she also suffered from impaired cognition. She had trouble thinking and sometimes was unable to express herself clearly.

Prior to her illness, Agnes was able to go into business meetings with little preparation—she was great at thinking on her feet. Now she needed a week to prepare and relied on extensive written notes to guide her through a meeting.

Before long, Agnes's business declined to the point that she nearly lost her livelihood. She no longer had the mental acuity needed to compete in a rapidly changing business environment. Seeing her assets dwindling, she became anxious and depressed. When Agnes first consulted with me, she told me that conducting business had become like "trying to work through a fog."

In addition to her diminished mental function, Agnes suffered from noticeable tremors in her arms and hands. Her voice, once vibrant and strong, had become weak. Her face had developed a "Parkinsonian mask" that made her appear listless.

Agnes's symptoms and her anxieties about their effect on her business became a vicious cycle, the mental stress exacerbating her tremors. She had the appearance of being nervous and weak, which put her at a distinct disadvantage in the high-level meetings she had to attend.

Within a week of her first stem cell treatment, Agnes's mind started to clear. After three weeks, she reported that her mental acuity was mostly restored, but that she was still experiencing tremors.

Three months later, Agnes's voice had regained its normal strength, and she took to conducting business over the phone as much as possible, so that clients wouldn't notice the tremors in her hands. Her trembling was noticeably improved, but she was still concerned about anyone misinterpreting her residual shaking as a sign of weakness. Her existing venture returned to profitability; she also launched a new branch of her business. She had become her former, successful, hard-driving self.

Today, Agnes's tremors are minimal—indeed, barely noticeable. She reports that she is back to business as usual and once more at the top of her field and is excited about her future.

Broderick

Broderick is a retired physician who had been suffering from Parkinson's disease for 15 years when I met him. He tried everything medically available to deal with his condition, including deep brain stimulation surgery, to no avail.

He was in an advanced stage of Parkinson's, having great difficulty walking and keeping his balance. His face had the rigid, lifeless aspect of the "Parkinsonian mask."

Broderick's cognitive abilities had deteriorated to the point that he couldn't pursue his passion for reading and study. According to his wife, Broderick had become depressed and withdrew from his family to the point that he barely spoke to her or their children.

In a follow-up report, Broderick's wife wrote the following:

A little over four months after Broderick received the cells, he was already walking almost normally and smiling again. He hasn't smiled for over two and a half years! His face is back to normal and his hands are much steadier.

His cognition has increased tremendously. He has begun studying calculus, biology, and physics, and is absorbed in reading books on these subjects. Books, in many cases, he hadn't touched in years, because he wasn't able to follow along with what he was reading.

He is also once again actively conversing and participating with our family and friends. The other day our daughter, who is a neurologist, examined him and told me that although she was unaware of ever experiencing or even knowing about such changes in a patient with Parkinson's, her father had definite and objectively tangible, meaningful improvements.

Alice, another of my patients, described very well what I think has been the experience of many of my Parkinson's patients:

"Every day is better than the last. I'm managing the Parkinson's disease instead of it managing me."

I must emphasize that the patients whose stories I have presented here experienced greater and more rapid improvements than are typical. I included some of the more dramatic cases to demonstrate the potential of the fetal stem cell treatment.

My father developed Parkinson's disease when I was a teenager. Before the disease took hold of him, he was very bright and active, a man to whom everyone turned whenever they had a problem. He was greatly respected in our community, very successful in business, and my mother's "knight in shining armor." I don't remember my parents ever fighting. They had their disagreements, but never for a moment did they lose their mutual love and respect for each other.

Soon after his first symptoms appeared, my father began to realize he could no longer function cognitively or physically as he had in the past. Before his illness, my father had been my mother's protector and caretaker. Now their roles had reversed and she was taking care of him. No matter how hard she tried, my mother was unable to hide her anguish and concern for him and although being ill was obviously not his fault, my father still felt very guilty that he was letting her down.

My father started to disappear, so to speak. He became increasingly depressed and withdrawn, to the point that, not wanting to become more of a burden to his loving wife, I believe he purposely created his own need to be hospitalized.

Eventually my father shut down completely, and soon thereafter he died. He was only 56 years old.

Sickle-Cell Anemia

Sickle-cell anemia is a hereditary disease that affects 70,000 Americans. It occurs when a child inherits two abnormal genes, one from each parent. People who inherit the sickle-cell gene from only one parent will not develop the disease, but they can pass the gene on to their children. The National Institutes of Health (NIH) recommends that newborn babies be screened for the sickle-cell gene.

Sickle-cell anemia affects the ability of red blood cells to carry oxygen to specific areas of the body. Normal red blood cells are round in shape. The red blood cells of a sickle-cell patient are abnormal in shape, resembling a crescent moon or a sickle. Unlike normal red blood cells, which move easily through even the smallest blood vessels, the abnormally shaped sickle cells can become stuck in the narrow blood vessels, thereby interfering with the transport of oxygen to cells, tissues, and organs.

Symptoms of sickle-cell anemia include extreme weakness, chronic fatigue, episodes of generalized extreme pain, and frequent serious bacterial infections.

Unlike normal red blood cells that live in the bloodstream for approximately four months, the fragile sickle cells usually deteriorate within 10 to 20 days. This accelerated breakdown of the sickle cells results in jaundice.

Also, sickle cells can become trapped in the lungs, causing severe chest and abdominal pain, fever, cough, and marked difficulty in breathing. Many children with sickle-cell anemia will not live beyond their teenage years.

Currently, most recommended treatments only help manage symptoms and prevent complications. They include pain medications, antibiotics, oxygen therapy and blood transfusions. At times, a splenectomy (removal of the spleen) is performed because the spleen, which filters the blood, is the principal organ in which the sickle cells get caught (splenic sequestration).

Aside from these palliative treatments, the only recognized therapy for sickle-cell anemia is a bone marrow transplant, but this is viable for only a very limited number of patients because of the difficulty of finding a donor match, the harmful side-effects of the required immunosuppressive drugs and the danger of graft-versus-host disease, wherein the donor cells attack the recipient.

The few cases of a reported positive intervention with a bone marrow transplant in patients with sickle-cell anemia involved identical twins, one of whom has the disease while the other does not. (Though it may seem unlikely, this can happen; identical twins are not entirely identical genetically). In these cases, the twin who has sickle-cell anemia is given a bone marrow transplant using bone marrow from the healthy twin. Even with twins, however, the bone marrow transplant required the use of both chemotherapy and dangerous immunosuppressive drugs, and it still carries the risk of graft-versus-host disease.

I have had the opportunity to treat two patients with sickle-cell anemia. My initial thought before treating them was, since fetal stem cells have greater than normal oxygen-carrying capacity, they might relieve the devastating symptoms of sickle-cell anemia. That is exactly what happened.

Marcus

My first sickle cell patient was a five-year-old boy named Marcus, who had been diagnosed with the disease at birth. He had suffered from constant infections, fevers, and severe generalized pain all his life. Consequently, he could not engage in the normal activities of children his age and could attend school only sporadically.

His parents had been told by their hematologist physician that Marcus would likely continue to suffer for the rest of his shorter than normal life.

A pre-treatment laboratory test (hemoglobin electrophoresis) showed that 96 percent of his red blood cells were sickle cells.

Marcus received only one fetal stem cell treatment. Within days, his symptoms began to reverse, and soon after, he became completely free of pain, his frequent chronic infections, and fevers.

Two months after treatment, Marcus was far more energetic; he returned to school full-time and joined his friends in normal childhood activities.

Six months after treatment, re-testing revealed that Marcus now had a significant level of fetal hemoglobin, a highly effective oxygen carrier, and that his sickle-cell hemoglobin count had dropped from 96 percent to 62 percent.

Marcus's recovery was so dramatic that it actually generated a complaint from his mother. A few weeks after he was treated she called me to say: "Everything is wonderful, except that Marcus seems to have become hyperactive. He's carrying on almost like he's out of control!"

I explained that Marcus's behavior was quite normal under the circumstances. He was like someone who had been unfairly imprisoned for most of his life, and then suddenly freed. Liberated from pain and illness, Marcus was excited to the point of appearing hyperactive as he discovered all the things he now was able to do, including actively playing with his friends. He was thrilled and making up for lost time. I assured her that he would settle down before long, which indeed he did.

It has been over nine years since Marcus received his single fetal stem cell treatment. He has no symptoms of sickle-cell anemia and is leading a normal, healthy, active life.

Such a benign intervention and sustained recovery have never been reported before in the medical literature.

Flora

My second sickle-cell patient, Flora, was 62 years old when I met her. Her doctors had told her that given the severity of her symptoms, she would at best live for one more year. Flora was in pain a great deal of the time and extremely thin. Due to an extreme lack of energy, she had great difficulty walking, and all of her movements were very slow.

Like Marcus, Flora received only one fetal stem cell treatment, and her symptoms soon began to reverse. Within a few weeks, she had markedly fewer painful episodes and was more energetic. She remained in this improved state until her death more than seven years later.

At the time Flora died, she was the oldest known sickle-cell patient in her country.

Marcus and Flora are the only sickle-cell patients that I have been able to treat so far. They both lived outside the United States.

When the chief hematologist in the country where they lived learned of their treatment with the fetal stem cells, he became infuriated—in spite of their successful recoveries.

I had scheduled a treatment for a third sickle-cell patient, a seven-year-old girl named Judy. The aforementioned hematologist learned of her scheduled treatment a week before it was to take place. He contacted Judy's mother and told her that the fetal stem cells could kill her child and then added that if she went ahead with the treatment, he would refuse to treat Judy ever again.

Judy's mother reported this conversation to us and said she had decided not to go forward. I made a number of attempts to discuss the matter with the hematologist. He refused to speak to me.

Judy remained in pain, with multiple infections that kept her from ever experiencing a normal child's life.

Judy died three years later, at the age of 10.

Stroke

Every 45 seconds someone in the United States has a stroke. **A quarter of them will die within the first year.**

It is the most common cause of adult disability in the United States, and the third most common cause of death, behind heart disease and cancer.

According to the Center for Disease Control (CDC) Stroke will cost the United States about $74 billion in 2010.

Stroke is defined as damage to a part of the brain caused by a lack of oxygen due to decreased blood flow. The brain is more sensitive to such damage than any other organ. The result of a stroke is the loss or impairment of whatever function is controlled by the damaged portion of the brain.

Stroke symptoms commonly include slurred speech, aphasia (total inability to speak), impairment or loss of vision, dizziness, headaches, difficulty swallowing, confusion, loss of motor control, and partial or complete paralysis.

A major cause of stroke is arteriosclerosis, the hardening and narrowing of the arteries, caused by plaque build-up on the arterial walls. When arteriosclerosis occurs in the cerebral arteries—which supply oxygen to the brain—the resulting decrease in blood flow significantly increases the risk of a stroke. Embolism, another common cause of stroke, occurs when an embolus—a blot clot migrating through the blood stream—lodges in the brain, blocking the blood supply. A less common cause of stroke is a ruptured blood vessel bleeding into the brain.

Modern medicine holds that there is a window of opportunity of only about six hours in which medical intervention can be of significant help to stroke victims. It is commonly accepted that after six hours, little can be done to significantly restore lost brain function, although some stroke victims do show some gradual improvement over time via the body's own reparative systems.

The improvements my patients have experienced, even years after their strokes, would be dismissed by most medical experts as unheard of and impossible.

George

One such patient is George, the police officer I wrote about earlier who had suffered a severe stroke two years before his daughter, a medical student, brought him to see me.

After George received his fetal stem cell treatment, his daughter wrote the following:

I was living the best years of my life before my father had his stroke. It was the last thing that I would have expected to happen to my active, vibrant, strong father.

As a result of the stroke, the left side of his body was almost completely non-functional, diminished by at least 85 percent, resulting in his left arm and leg becoming virtually useless. His speech was also severely affected, to the point that we were barely able to understand him. His vision was also severely impaired.

Besides the physiological consequences, my father was emotionally devastated. He became very depressed and, at times, very angry and aggressive. Having been a policeman, being physically active and healthy all of his life, you can imagine what this illness meant for him. It was like the end of his world. Most of the time, all he did was lie in bed murmuring that he was never going to be the man he used to be again.

That all changed after he received the fetal stem cells. Despite two years of progressive deterioration, my father experienced a nearly instantaneous recovery. As he was receiving the cells, his speech and vision began to clear. At first these changes actually made him angry, because he wasn't nearly as concerned about his diminished speech and vision, compared to how much he wanted to regain the use of his arm and leg. He started to become upset with me, thinking I had brought him to a doctor who had given him the wrong treatment. But then he calmed down, once Dr. Rader and I explained to him that this was just the initial change, and the cells he received would, hopefully, eventually also restore function in his arm and leg.

In the first week after my father received the fetal stem cells, his attitude changed noticeably for the better. He was far more enthusiastic about life and took an active role in his recovery by working with a physical therapist. The therapist and I were both impressed, because previously, depressed and resigned to his fate, he had adamantly refused to consider physical therapy or any other form of help. One week later, the physical therapist reported that my father was becoming much more flexible and was exhibiting many other positive changes that left her shocked, because we hadn't told her about the stem cell treatment.

As I write this second letter, 12 weeks from the time of his treatment, there are considerable, noticeable changes still occurring in my father's recovery. His mobility has increased by 70 percent and his speech is almost perfect—99 percent recovered!

Two years after his first treatment (four years after his stroke), George requested a second fetal stem cell treatment. In a follow-up report, his daughter wrote:

My father tells me he that he now has so much energy that he is going nonstop. He says he feels as if he is receiving positive electric charges in his arm and leg and that in general his entire body has been revitalized. The positive changes just continue to surge through him. His walking is now just about normal, and he is driving!

Last week when I saw him after being away in medical school I started crying because I couldn't believe what I was seeing.

In addition, my mother told me she is very happy about the stem cell treatment because his abilities in intimate activities are better than ever—if you know what I mean. She is even asking me if my father can possibly get more cells!

Without a doubt, the fetal stem cells have changed my life in numerous ways. And obviously my father's and mother's lives as well!

Phillip

Phillip's stroke left him with significantly impaired vision and slurred speech. The left side of his mouth drooped. His poor balance made walking difficult.

Before coming to me, Phillip had received umbilical cord stem cells. He told me that this treatment had yielded "no significant results."

He was understandably skeptical about stem cell treatment in general, and unsure whether fetal stem cells could help him.

I understood his reluctance and suggested he should read as much as could about stem cells and get back to me with any questions. We had many conversations, with Phillip asking multiple questions based on his research. Eventually, he decided to proceed with the treatment.

Less than 45 minutes after Phillip received the fetal stem cells, he reported that he felt his vision had improved. According to his wife, within the next few hours, his speech was becoming clearer. The next day, his face became more symmetrical and his balance was improved. She told me, "Phillip has been laughing ecstatically, overjoyed at what was happening, when he had previously lost all hope that he could ever recover."

Why did fetal stem cells make a difference for Philip after treatment with umbilical cells yielded no significant improvement? Both stem cell therapies use hematopoietic (blood) stem cells, but fetal stem cell therapy has two main advantages. It provides the most powerful kind of hematopoietic stem cell. Furthermore, the patient receives a vital second type of stem cell not found in umbilical cord cells—a neuronal (nerve) stem cell obtained from the brain of the fetus. This neuronal stem cell is essential in the treatment of stroke, as well as for other neurological diseases.

Other stroke patients have reported reversal of hearing loss, significant increases in energy, healthy weight gain, better memory (most significantly in short-term memory), and other improvements.

Although most of the stroke patients treated with the fetal stem cells, in general have had marked improvements, each individual patient's outcome is different. A minor number of them have experienced only a limited gain in function.

If fetal stem cells were to be stored in liquid nitrogen aboard ambulances, so that they could be administered by emergency response teams to stroke patients within those critical first six hours, the devastating effects of a patient's stroke would be significantly reduced— and in many cases, completely eliminated.

My Hope

If the truth can be told so as to be understood, it will be believed.

—Terence McKenna, paraphrasing William Blake

I have three main purposes in writing this book.

The first is to offer hope to the hopeless. When people are told that there is no hope for their recovery, or for their children's, I want them to know that fetal stem cell therapy exists.

To have the "experts" understand what it is and how it can benefit mankind.

Lastly, I would like everyone to have a choice that mainstream medicine won't even mention much less offer.

I expect some of my readers to remain skeptical. They want to know—as they should—why I haven't published my data in a prominent American medical journal.

I've answered that question throughout this book, but I feel it bears repeating. No mainstream medical journal will publish results not based on extensive double-blind studies. I didn't become interested in fetal stem cells out of scholarly curiosity. I became impassioned over their use after I saw with my own eyes some of the recoveries of those patients in the Ukraine in 1995.

I guess I could have chosen to push for an animal research project that could eventually pave the way for human trials and then perhaps bring fetal stem cell therapy into approved use for humans 20 years later. Instead, I decided to put this therapy into use for human patients right away, because my instincts and my morality would not allow me to wait.

I am not willing to be patient and stand still in the face of death and suffering—or the inertia of bureaucracy, the fear and greed of vested interests, and the prejudices of the intellectually indolent.

My patients don't have the luxury of time. They need help now. So I'll keep on treating them and continue to devote my best efforts to sharing with the rest of the medical world what I have learned.

Following publication of this book I will, as I've said, make all my data available for review and study. If I am a quack and a fraud and this book is a pack of lies, then my critics will have every chance to expose me once and for all.

But if diligent, objective examination of my data and my patients' case histories confirms what I have told you, then I need your help. If you believe in the potential of this treatment, please join me in advocating that fetal stem cell therapy be legitimized and made available in the United States, or at least that human trials begin as soon as possible.

If fetal stem cells were legalized in the United States I would become able to actualize multiple theories I have regarding methods of new treatments. For example for a spinal cord injury patient performing a neurosurgical procedure in which the damaged area of the spinal cord is removed and put in its place is a biodegradable matrix *(a framework which is eventually absorbed by the body)*. The neuronal fetal stem cells would then be placed throughout the structure creating new nerve cells which will then grow and attach themselves to both ends of the open cord. The result would be the spinal cord now being intact having the ability to transmit messages from the brain to the rest of the body.

If fetal stem cells were legalized in the United States we would have thousands of doctors, scientists and researchers starting where I am now. No matter how smart I may be I am only one person. Now imagine what could be accomplished by all that scientific manpower and billions of dollars. At best I and my scientific team have been able to create a horse and buggy. Man has gotten to the moon.

This is a fight for human progress, and for many it is a fight for life. At the very least, my work deserves to be fairly evaluated. And above all, my patients deserve to have their voices heard.

Thank you for hearing them.

About The Author

William C. Rader, M.D. is the only American physician involved in the actual clinical application of human fetal stem cells. Since 1995 he has successfully treated more than 1,500 patients.

Dr. Rader earned his medical degree with honors from the State University of New York at Buffalo in 1967, and was first in his psychiatric residency class at the University of Southern California Medical Center in 1971.

Dr. Rader served as chief psychiatrist for the U.S. Navy's alcoholic treatment program from 1971 to 1973. He developed a widely used training program for alcoholism counselors.

His family system approach, a successful mental health treatment model that empowered individuals to achieve and then maintain their recovery from addiction, was adopted as an integral part of the Betty Ford recovery program at the Eisenhower Medical Center in Rancho Mirage, California.

He is recognized as a pioneer in the fields of alcoholism, drug addiction, eating disorders (bulimia, anorexia, and compulsive overeating), codependency, sexual addiction, sexual abuse and most recently stem cell clinical research.

Dr. Rader's accomplishments include:

Founded

- The Rader Institute (1984). The world's largest eating disorder treatment program. Not focused on weight loss, it was specifically tailored for patients suffering from anorexia, bulimia and compulsive overeating.

- The Survivor Program (1992). Identifying sexual abuse victims as having a distinct disorder requiring specialized treatment. Helping victims of sexual abuse become empowered survivors

- The Immune Suppressed Institute Mexico City, Mexico (1993) one of the first HIV/AIDS treatment centers in Latin America.

- Medra Inc (1995), an international corporation dedicated to the research and development of the clinical application of fetal stem cells.

Research

- Chief International Research Consultant for Columbia Laboratories, one of Mexico's largest pharmaceutical companies. His research included a project involving a benign combination of amino acids which significantly reduced atherosclerotic plaque (beginning 1993).

- State University Medical School at Buffalo. In vivo preparation of kidneys for transplantation.

Featured lecturer

- The American Psychiatric Association.

- The Annual Symposium on Addictive Disorders.

- The National Eating Disorders Association Annual Conference.

Publications

- The Journal of the American Medical Association (JAMA).

About The Author

Membership

- American Medical Association (AMA).
- California Medical Association (CMA).

Awards

- Honors. State University at Buffalo Medical School (1967).
- The Sandoz Award (first in his psychiatric residency class, USC, 1971)
- Naval Commendation for his service as the chief psychiatrist of the Naval alcohol treatment program.
- Overeaters Anonymous (1982 Man of the Year).
- The National Council on Alcoholism.
- Emmy Los Angeles "Rape The Hidden Crime."

Dr. Rader has been the only American physician researching the therapeutic applications of fetal stem cell therapy. In 1995 he founded Medra Inc., an international corporation dedicated to the research and development of the clinical application of fetal stem cells. He currently serves as chairman of the board, medical director, and chief scientist.

Media

- Appearances - Dr. Rader appeared on television as a medical expert for more than a decade.
  - Serving as a medical expert for ABC television's "Good Morning America.".
  - Appeared twice weekly from 1977 to 1991 as a medical expert for KABC Eyewitness News in Los Angeles.

- Served as a medical expert for WABC Eyewitness News in New York.

- Appeared weekly as their medical expert on the nationally syndicated television programs "Hour Magazine," and "The Home Show".

- He was a regular guest on "Donahue," "Jenny Jones," "Leeza,", "Montel Williams" and "The Sally Jesse Raphael Show," shedding new light on important medical, psychological, and social issues, some of which had never before been explored on television

- Producer

  - Produced television shows, selecting the guests and co-hosting programs for "Geraldo," "The Mike Douglas Show," "The Merv Griffin Show," and "The Tomorrow Show" with Tom Snyder. When TV Guide reviewed "The Tomorrow Show," they cited Dr. Rader's program as one of the two best episodes in the program's history. When Newsweek reviewed all TV talk shows of that period, they praised the episodes of "The Merv Griffin Show" that Dr. Rader had co-hosted and produced.

- Writer

  - Wrote an episode of "All In The Family" in which Archie Bunker become addicted to diet pills. The groundbreaking episode demonstrated that diet pills, easily available by prescription, had a very serious addictive potential. The episode was submitted for an Emmy

o Wrote, produced and hosted numerous health-related documentaries for ABC.

o Book Dr. Rader's No Diet Program For Permanent Weight Loss

- Consultant
  o Technical advisor for television movies dealing with socially relevant issues.
  o NBC's "Sarah T: Portrait of a Teenage Alcoholic" (1975). It was the highest-rated TV movie of its season.
  o CBS's "Intimate Strangers" (1977) exposed the true nature of spousal abuse.

He also served as medical technical consultant for Paramount Studios, Tandem Productions and Universal Television.

References

[i] Fox, Cynthia, "Why Stem Cells Will Transform Medicine," Fortune Magazine online, June 11, 2001. http://money.cnn.com/magazines/fortune/fortune_archive/2001/06/11/304634/index.htm "Human stem cells promote healing of diabetic ulcer," University of Bristol circulation release

[ii] Israel21c staff, "Israeli scientists reverse brain defects using stem cells," Israel21c.org, December 25, 2008. http://www.israel21c.org/index.php?option=com_content&view=article&id=2296&catid=57:health&Itemid=63

[iii] Biotechnology and Biological Sciences Research Council, "Stem cells could help treat strokes," Kings College London web site, March 9, 2009. http://www.kcl.ac.uk/news/news_details.php?news_id=1023&year=2009

[iv] "Human stem cells promote healing of diabetic ulcer," University of Bristol circulation release paper, April 20, 2009. http://www.eurekalert.org/pub_releases/2009-04/uob-hsc042009.php

[v] Ray of Hope! Stem cell therapy 'to cure blindness,'" The Times of India web site, April 19, 2009. http://timesofindia.indiatimes.com/Health--Science/Science/Ray-of-Hope-Stem-cell-therapy-to-cure-blindness/articleshow/4420398.cms

[vi] "U Researcher Proves Potency of Tumor-Killing Cells from Human Embryonic Stem Cells," University of Minnesota Academic Health Center, May 4, 2009. http://www.ahc.umn.edu/news/releases/stemcells050409/home.html

[vii] Gucciardo, L. et al., "Fetal mesenchymal stem cells: isolation, properties and potential use in perinatology and regenerative medicine," National Center for Biological Information, January 2009. http://www.ncbi.nlm.nih.gov/pubmed/19076948

[viii] Jafarzadeh, Suad, "Iran at forefront of stem cell research," Washington Times online, April 15, 2009. http://www.washingtontimes.com/news/2009/apr/15/iran-at-forefront-of-stem-cell-research

[ix] Ritter, Malcolm, "US approves 1st stem cell study for spinal injury," SFGate, January 23, 2009. http://www.sfgate.com/cgi-bin/article.cgi?f=/n/a/2009/01/22/national/a210354S61.DTL&type=science

[x] Park, Alice, "Stem Cell Research: The Quiet Resumes," Time.com, January 29, 2009. http://www.time.com/time/health/article/0,8599,1874717-3,00.html

[xi] Russell, Sabin, "'Adult' stem cells could skirt embryos' ethical dilemmas," SFGate, June 25, 2005. http://www.sfgate.com/cgi-bin/article.cgi?file=/c/a/2005/06/25/MNGTKDF1LI1.DTL#ixzz0OUmWHLo8

[xii] Philipkoski, Kristin, "Fetal Cells Nix Rules, Fix Hearts," Wired.com, June 6, 2005. http://www.wired.com/medtech/health/news/2005/06/67763

[xiii] diverdonreed, "A Global Shout: How Will You Celebrate Stem Cell Awareness Day," Stem Cell Battles, July 15, 2009. http://stemcellbattles.wordpress.com/2009/07/15/a-global-shout-how-will-you-celebrate-stem-cell-awareness-day

[xiv] Stem cells could repair brain damage," BBC News Online, January 21, 2003. http://news.bbc.co.uk/2/hi/health/2673343.stm

[xv] Steenhuysen, Julie, "Doctors: Under the drug industry's influence?" Reuters.com, February 4, 2009. http://www.reuters.com/article/healthNews/idUSTRE5130ZZ20090204

[xvi] Kravchenko, Julia et al., "Endothelial Progenitor Cell Therapy for Atherosclerosis: The Philosopher's Stone for an Aging Population?" Science online, June 22, 2005. http://sageke.sciencemag.org/cgi/content/abstract/2005/25/pe18

[xvii] Randal, "Bone Marrow Stem Cell Aging Increases Leukemia and Infection Risks," FuturePundit.com, June 28, 2005. http://www.futurepundit.com/archives/002861.html

[xviii] Johnson, Lucy, "Have doctors discovered a cure for HIV?" Daily Express online, April 26, 2009. http://www.dailyexpress.co.uk/posts/view/97157

[xix] Schmidt, Elaine, "New compounds boost immune system's fight against HIV," University of California UC Newsroom, March 11, 2005. http://www.universityofcalifornia.edu/news/article/6996

[xx] Fiala, Milan et al., "Ineffective phagocytosis of amyloid-ß by macrophages of Alzheimer's disease patients," *Journal of Alzheimer's Disease*, Vol 7, number 3, June 2005. http://www.j-alz.com/issues/7/vol7-3.html